Caring for
Someone
with AIDS

Caring for Someone with AIDS

Edited by David Yelding

Published for the Research Institute for Consumer Affairs by Consumers' Association and Hodder & Stoughton

Caring for Someone with AIDS was commissioned and researched
by the Research Institute for Consumer Affairs, and published
by Consumers' Association, 2 Marylebone Road, London NW1 4DX
and Hodder & Stoughton, 47 Bedford Square, London WC1B 3DP

British Library Cataloguing in Publication Data

Caring for Someone with AIDS
  1. AIDS patients. Care
  I. Yelding, David   II. Consumers' Association
  362.1969792

ISBN 0 340 52678 5

Edited by David Yelding

Contributors
Andrew Armstrong, Journalist
David Bickerton, Former Drugs Counselling Officer, Terrence Higgins Trust
Anna Bradley, Research Manager, Consumers' Association
Ginny Bruce, Researcher
John Church, Carers Service Co-ordinator, St Mary's Hospital, Paddington
Michael Dunne, MBE, BSc, Disablement Income Group
Duncan Guthrie, OBE, LLD, MA, Director, Disabilities Study Unit
Jacqueline Hockings, BSc, MSc, CQSW, Former Counselling Officer, Terrence Higgins Trust
Agnes Kocsis, Senior Clinical Psychologist, St Mary's Hospital, Paddington
Jeni McCallion, BA, (Hons) Law, of Lincoln's Inn, Barrister
Kate Skinner, Former AIDS Advisor, Lothian Region Social Work Department
Dr Ian Williams, BSc, MRCP(UK), Middlesex Hospital

Text design by Peter Kneebone
Cover design by Paul Saunders

Phototypesetting by Paston Press, Loddon, Norfolk
Printed and bound in Great Britain by the Bath Press, Bath

RICA and the Disabilities Study Unit gratefully acknowledge funding from the Department of
Health, Leigh Trust, The Monument Trust, and also The Goodhart Charitable Trust, The G S
Sanders Charitable Settlement and The Thorn Trust.

Contents

Introduction   9
What is AIDS?   11
  How is HIV transmitted?
  Stages of infection

Caring   19
  First thoughts
  Living with AIDS and being in control
  About carers
  Some key points

Help, information and services   47
  Finding out what's available
  Help through doctors
  Help through social workers
  Services set up for people with AIDS
  Hospices
  Other voluntary organisations
  Taking things further

Counselling   83
  What is counselling?
  How to find a counsellor
  Psychotherapy
  Clinical psychologists
  Family therapy
  Other sources of help

Legal matters   93
    Power of attorney
    Life insurance
    Employment
    Help with legal costs
    Making a will
    More information

Home nursing   109

Housing   121
    Finding accommodation
    Housing law
    Adaptations

Transport   137

Cash help   143
    Social security and other benefits
    Special funds and charities

Symptoms and medical treatment   185
    Symptoms
    Current treatment
    Anti-HIV treatment

Complementary medicine   199

Partners and families   203
    Caring for a partner
    Families

Pregnancy and children   213
    Pregnancy
    Caring for children
    Care and guardianship
    Help and advice

Drug users and HIV   225
    Some basic guidelines
    Sources of help
    Addresses

Haemophilia   245

When someone dies   247

Bereavement   255

Religious and spiritual support   263

Caring for the carer   267
  Ways of making caring easier
  Stress
  Support for carers
  Taking time off

Appendices   289
  Booklist
  Safer sex
  Safer drugs
  Local helplines
  Feedback

Index   305

Introduction

AIDS has been a challenge for many of us. It has challenged the medical profession to find new methods of treatment and eventually a cure. It has challenged our views about sexuality and sexual behaviour. It has challenged statutory and voluntary agencies to find ways of meeting new demands. Carers – partners, families, friends and professional staff have been confronted by an overwhelming number of issues. But the greatest challenges have been faced by individual people with AIDS.

At first people with AIDS had to cope with the devastating consequences of an illness about which very little was known. Enormous difficulties were caused by widespread misinformation and prejudice. But in this unpromising terrain has grown the strength, courage, humour and grace to fight back.

Not all the battles have been won. Prejudice still persists, and services for people with AIDS are patchy. However, the number and variety of organisations described in this book show how much has been achieved in building systems of practical support and sources of inspiration and encouragement.

Most people want to make their own decisions and direct their own lives. Although this book is dedicated to carers we stress that this does not suggest that the carer should assume all responsibility. How responsibilities are shared and how matters are to be sorted out will depend on the wishes of the person with AIDS, individual relationships and many other personal considerations. So the 'you' we address in this book may be the person with AIDS or it may be a partner, relative, friend or anyone who is asked to help.

There is no right or wrong way of living with AIDS. This book cannot lay down rules. It describes some of the situations and concerns you may be faced with and suggests some possible ways of dealing with them. It is worth emphasising that AIDS is not something which has to be faced alone. One of the challenges which has been met in a spectacular way is the call for mutual support. Many self-help groups have been set up – they are approachable, friendly, understanding, well informed and generous. They are likely to be your greatest asset.

This book covers a lot of ground. Don't be daunted by this. It is mostly a directory of resources to be used where and when appropriate. No one will want it all.

Many people with AIDS have managed to remain well for long periods, and have not needed any of the sort of help we describe. Indeed, many have found that it has provided them with an opportunity to review their lives and find ways of developing new interests and spending time in a more rewarding way.

Our thanks go to the very many people who contributed information to this book, read and commented on drafts and made helpful suggestions. In particular we would like to thank the people with AIDS, their carers, families and friends who talked to us during the research; some of their thoughts and experiences appear throughout the book.

NOTE: for simplicity we usually use 'AIDS' very broadly to include both ARC and AIDS itself. Where it is sensible to distinguish between them we do so. Unless we say otherwise we use HIV or HIV infection to include those who are HIV-positive as well as people with ARC or AIDS. See chapter 1 for more information about all these.

1

What is AIDS?

In this chapter we explain what HIV, ARC and AIDS are and give a simplified account of what is now known about them. In Chapter 10 we describe some common symptoms and give information about the treatments available, some of the medical terms used, and the names of some of the drugs in current use, in case you come across these in dealing with hospital or medical staff.

You need to know and understand as much as you can about the diagnosis and treatment. Don't be afraid to ask questions. When you get different answers from different people ask them to explain. But bear in mind that much is still unknown and that there may be some questions which can't be answered conclusively. A great deal of research is under way and knowledge and theories about HIV illnesses and their treatment is constantly changing. See page 295 for how to get up-to-date information.

In the early 1980s doctors in the USA began seeing an unusual respiratory infection and a rare form of skin cancer called Kaposi's sarcoma (KS) in young gay men. All the men were found to have a damaged immune system (the body's built-in mechanism for fighting disease). In 1983 in France and in 1984 in the USA researchers isolated a virus as the cause. This was eventually named as the Human Immunodeficiency Virus 1. (Since then another related virus, HIV II, has been found and experts believe other forms may be discovered. Throughout this book we have used HIV to include all strains of the virus.)

A virus is a very simple living organism, consisting of a capsule containing genetic material. It can live and reproduce only inside a living cell in the body. There are many different viruses which, by invading particular types of cell, cause diseases such as the common cold and polio. Once inside, the virus literally takes the cell over, using it as a factory to produce more viruses. In turn, these leave the parent cell and go on to infect new cells.

The HIV virus grows in *T-helper cells* which are essential to the normal function of the immune system. So when T-helper cells infected with HIV eventually die, the immune system is seriously damaged. As a result of this people become susceptible to unusual infections and tumours. This is called the *Acquired Immune Deficiency Syndrome* or AIDS.

How is HIV transmitted?

The virus can survive only by colonising individual cells in the body. You can become infected if cells containing it enter your own body. The virus is so far known to spread by certain kinds of sexual contact, by blood, from infected sperm in donor insemination and from mother to baby.

Sexual contact

In Europe and North America, most of those who have been diagnosed so far as having AIDS are either gay or bisexual men. But AIDS can affect anybody. In 'first world' countries the gay communities happen to have experienced it first. In other parts of the world such as Africa, where AIDS is much more common than in Britain, the virus seems to have spread mostly as a result of heterosexual sex.

Experts don't know precisely how the virus is transmitted sexually. One theory is that semen and vaginal fluids may infect the membranes lining the vagina or rectum and the skin covering the penis.

But, whatever the explanation, it is clear from the pattern of the spread of HIV throughout the world that it can be transmitted by either anal or vaginal sexual intercourse, and that it can be passed on from a man to woman or to another man, and from a woman to a man. Other sexual practices are much less risky. Oral sex may carry a small risk; otherwise, most sexual activities are safe – see the appendix for more information on safer sex.

Blood

Infected blood has to get into your bloodstream for infection by blood to be possible. The virus can be transmitted during the transfusion of contaminated blood or blood products or through an operation (such as a transplant or skin graft) if the donor was infected.

However, there is now virtually no risk in the UK of infection occurring by means of transmission by blood other than by sharing syringes and needles with infected people. Since 1986 people in 'high risk groups' and those known to be infected are asked not to give blood or donate organs. Today all blood donated in Europe or the USA is checked for HIV antibodies. (Tests for HIV-2, the virus now known to be responsible for many cases of AIDS in West Africa, may be introduced if HIV-2 looks like spreading to this country.)

There remains an extremely small risk that a recently infected person who gives blood has not yet produced antibodies to HIV (see below under Stages of infection, Stage I) and, therefore, goes undetected. It is hoped that in the future new tests for the virus itself, not just the antibodies, will be available so even this minute risk will be eliminated. Blood products, for example the clotting factor that haemophiliacs need, are treated to kill any virus that may be present. There is no need to fear having a blood transfusion or organ transplant now.

However, drug users can become infected with HIV if they share needles or syringes with another drug user who is already infected. Research shows that most injecting drug users share needles at some stage.

Infection by blood in any other, less direct, way is unlikely. It is possible only if the skin is broken – for example if you have a new cut or wound. There have been a few cases in the USA where the disease has been transmitted in this way. However, even a cut that's only a few hours old would develop a protective layer which would stop the virus. Any small risk can be avoided by taking normal precautions to avoid any kind of infection when clearing up someone else's blood.

Donor insemination	The risk of infection through donated sperm is now negligible. The Department of Health recommends that donors are tested for HIV infection at the time of donation and that semen is frozen until a second blood test three months later. Use of freshly donated semen may pose a greater risk because HIV tests may not show up a recent infection.
Birth	If a mother is infected by HIV before or during her pregnancy there is a chance that her baby will also carry the virus. See page 214 for more information.
Myths and risks	There has been much misinformation about the risks of HIV infection, sometimes leading to totally unjustified discrimination – refusing to work with an HIV-positive colleague, and refusing to allow children to attend a school which has an HIV-positive pupil are examples. But, as we have explained above, the HIV virus is quite difficult to catch. It is readily destroyed by household bleach.
Sharing a household	Studies of family and friends who live with an infected person have shown there is no risk of becoming infected as a result of normal family contact, towels, cutlery, crockery, drinking glasses and lavatories.
Kissing	The quantity of virus that is sometimes found in saliva or tears is minute in comparison with the amount found in semen, vaginal fluid or blood, and experts think that you generally need to come into contact with substantial amounts of the virus to become infected. The only conceivable risk from saliva exchange is with intimate 'French' or wet kissing, but experts think that even this presents virtually no risk.
Caring and nursing	Even hospital staff who come into very close contact with people with HIV become infected extremely rarely. Several hundred health workers are known to have pricked themselves with a needle used to treat someone with HIV and yet there are only two cases of British health workers becoming infected in this way. There is very little risk of becoming infected by HIV by caring for someone with AIDS, and even this can be eliminated by very simple precautions. On page 119 we describe the basic rules of hygiene when nursing someone who is ill.

It is not possible to be infected with HIV by:

- being bitten by insects
- sharing a bathroom or toilet with an infected person
- sharing an ordinary working or social environment with an infected person
- touching an infected person
- breathing the same air as an infected person
- handling money
- sharing the same equipment – crockery, cutlery, stationery, furniture etc. as an infected person
- using the same swimming pool or shower as an infected person.

Stages of infection

The Centers for Disease Control (CDC) in the USA has divided the stages of HIV infection into four groups.

Stage I

Known as *acute infection*, this is when a person is first infected by the HIV virus. The majority of people have no symptoms at this stage and will look and feel well. Others experience an illness rather like glandular fever – symptoms which can occur are headaches, fever, chills, night sweats, rashes and temporary swelling of the lymph glands.

Those who have no symptoms will know that they are infected only if they have a blood test to see if they have developed antibodies to HIV. When someone starts to produce antibodies they are said to have seroconverted and be seropositive, HIV-positive, or antibody positive.

At the moment the main test for HIV infection is based on detecting antibodies to the virus. In most cases it takes up to three months before the immune system produces antibodies. So if a risk of infection is suspected in the last three months the test should be delayed or repeated to produce more definite results. However, recent evidence has suggested that some infected people may not produce antibodies for many months. A positive test result shows that a person has been infected by HIV. It doesn't mean they have AIDS, nor does it necessarily mean that they will develop AIDS in the future. They will, however, be infectious. It is possible that people are more infectious at two stages than at other times – between infection and the time when antibodies appear and when symptoms of an opportunistic infection are present (see below under Stage IV).

Stage II

No obvious symptoms develop during Stage II and those affected continue to be well. However, people who have been told that they are HIV-positive often suffer depression and anxiety as a consequence and may need expert counselling.

Stage III

The only symptom at this stage is persistent generalised lymphadenopathy (PGL). PGL is persistent swelling of the glands (under the jaw, in the neck, armpits or groin – all are also common symptoms of other diseases) for three months or more. Apart from this, people with PGL are well and are no more or less likely than those at Stage II to go on to develop AIDS itself.

Stage IV

Stage IV includes AIDS-Related Complex (ARC), AIDS itself and other complications due to HIV infection.

Many illnesses can develop at this stage, and many have severe and debilitating symptoms. Some are due to the direct effect of HIV infection, others to what are known as opportunistic infections and tumours which occur as a result of damage to the immune system.

AIDS-Related Complex (ARC) is the name given to a combination of symptoms including minor opportunistic infections (such as thrush or skin conditions) and specific general symptoms (such as chronic diarrhoea, fever or weight loss) which appear for three months or longer. In people with ARC the immune system has been weakened but usually less so than with AIDS. People with ARC are more susceptible to infections and other diseases, and are highly likely to go on to develop AIDS. Many of the symptoms common among people with ARC may also be symptoms of other diseases unrelated to HIV.

However, the diagnosis of ARC can cover anything from a mild case of thrush to severe debilitation or wasting. Symptoms can be similar to mild cases of HIV infection and more severe forms may be similar to AIDS itself.

People with AIDS have one or more specific diseases which reflect an underlying immune deficiency. The weakened system leaves the person open to opportunistic infections and tumours which would not otherwise occur, or be harmless. The most common are particular types of pneumonia, a form of skin tumour (Kaposi's sarcoma), thrush in the mouth, throat and gullet, persistent diarrhoea and certain forms of brain disease which cause convulsions, partial paralysis, blindness or dementia. Some can be treated successfully but for others the most that the treatment now available can do is to reduce their severity.

Although no one has yet been cured of AIDS, treatment has been shown to improve life expectancy and produce periods of relatively good health.

It was once thought that only a minority of people with HIV infection would go on to develop AIDS. It is now believed that at least half will develop AIDS within eight years of being infected. It is still too early to be certain what the final proportion may be, or how long AIDS may take to develop.

Estimates are based on what has happened in the past, and are usually based on studies of small samples of people. Future patterns may be different, particularly as treatment for HIV is improving and life expectancy is increasing. It is also impossible to say how any individual will be affected. Statistics show averages and probabilities, not what will happen to any one person.

Some people have developed AIDS within two years of being infected, while others still have not developed any symptoms years after being diagnosed as being HIV-positive. No one knows why some people with HIV infection develop AIDS and other don't. Theories about these differences have included the strength of different strains of HIV, the incidence of other infections (such as certain types of Herpes virus) and repeated exposure to the virus. Other possibilities are poor diet and heavy use of alcohol or drugs. As yet there is no conclusive evidence either way about any of these. Many people believe that the general health and attitude of the infected person may be the most important factor of all.

2 Caring

First thoughts

Caring is about being involved in life, and not endlessly contemplating death and its consequences

Caring is an intensely individual activity. Every relationship and every situation is different. There will be a great number of things which people with AIDS and those who are close to them can only work out together, or, if necessary, with the help of someone who can offer personal counselling. However, some basic guidelines, which emerged very strongly in our research, are worth stating at the beginning of the book.

The first is perhaps the most important. Don't fall into the trap of thinking that 'caring for someone' means taking over someone's life and making decisions for them. Your real aim should be to ensure that it is possible for the person with HIV to live in the way he or she wishes. What this help may consist of will depend on the person and his or her circumstances. At times you may be asked to take on a more decisive role and at others (during bouts of illness, say) you may *have* to do so. Alternatively, you may just be needed to help with minor practical tasks. You may even find that the best course of action is to do no more than be the same friend you have always been.

Having an HIV infection, or even being ill, does not mean that someone suddenly becomes unable to think or act independently. You should not intrude on anyone's right to control his or her own life.

> *Just be there and listen and try to support decisions. Let him know he's completely in control of his destiny*

> 'He's very supportive and doesn't make me feel incapable or an invalid. It's important to be able to think I'm actually a human being under all this'

Secondly, you both should try to get as much support as you need. Throughout this book we give details of organisations which may be able to help.

Many, particularly outside major cities, exist to help anyone who needs them, for whatever reason, not just to deal with problems related to HIV. Sometimes, their name or the way they describe themselves may seem inappropriate. For example, many organisations see themselves as providing services for people with disabilities. Don't let this put you off. All the information in this book has been checked with the organisations listed. We have not included any which have nothing to offer people with HIV or their carers, although some are very stretched.

However, it is unfortunately still true that some people are prejudiced, ignorant and frightened or turn out to be unsympathetic. For this reason it is worth sounding out any local group or person before you approach them. If you do come across people who are difficult it is worth taking the matter up with the organiser or head office of the organisation concerned. AIDS organisations may also be interested to know what happens.

Finally, it is worth saying that HIV, ARC and AIDS are unpredictable. People who are HIV-positive may remain in good health for long periods – perhaps indefinitely. They will need few, if any, of the services and facilities described in this book. People with ARC or AIDS may or may not develop any of the opportunistic illnesses described in chapter 10. Some people remain relatively healthy, and experience comparatively minor complaints. Some have periods of sickness followed by periods of good health. Some may develop various symptoms simultaneously and need fairly intensive care. But even people who become very ill can make a strong recovery.

As medical treatment continues to get better, people are remaining healthy for longer. It is not possible to know in advance what may happen. Try not to be overwhelmed by the thought of what may lie ahead. Take things as they come.

Living with AIDS and being in control

We have explained how one of your main tasks as a carer may be to help the person with AIDS stay in control of his or her own life. This section describes some of the ways people with AIDS have found of doing so. For more information see the booklist on page 289.

A diagnosis of AIDS does not mean an end to living, but for many people it does mean dramatic changes. They may experience appalling feelings of loss, pain and anger but many people have also found new beginnings. Some have reported that the changes AIDS has forced on their lives have been for the better. There is no right or wrong way to cope with AIDS. There is only an individual way, which will be different for each person. Some strategies that people with AIDS have developed are outlined below.

Think and act positively

Believing that AIDS is not an immediate death sentence takes strength and energy. The person with AIDS has to be convinced that he or she is in control rather than the virus, which can be difficult because so many circumstances seem to conspire against this. Doctors and hospitals can 'take over' and address the symptoms to be treated rather than the person. Some people find they are regarded as 'patients' who need to be managed and have decisions taken for them.

> One of the most important things for people with this illness is to maintain their own power. People used not to fight . . .

Fighting can take many forms. Some people collect information so they can discuss or argue with doctors over methods of treatment. Others find that it helps to set targets to achieve (seeing people, joining a support group, learning a new skill, for example). Some become aware of the gaps in services for people with AIDS and join or initiate campaigns to change things. All such strategies help to dissipate feelings of helplessness, which can be overwhelming, particularly in the early stages after diagnosis. Many people have been surprised at the new skills they have developed to meet the challenge they faced.

Any action can help get rid of the feeling that HIV is an uncertain, unpredictable enemy which can only be reacted to. It *is* rather unpredictable but no one should just sit and wait passively for the worst.

Take time to make decisions

Once the initial shock of being HIV-positive has lessened it is possible to make plans for the future. Decisions have to be made about every aspect of life – about medical treatment, about work, about staying in a relationship, and so on. This takes careful thought and involves considering a huge number of issues.

It is usually best not to make radical choices too quickly, especially in the first couple of months after someone has been diagnosed as being HIV-positive. There is so much going on that it may be difficult to believe that there will be time to talk over any major decisions with close friends, but ideas should be allowed to settle before they are put into action.

Think about priorities

Being diagnosed as HIV-positive means that things that once mattered may no longer seem important, and things once thought trivial become significant. Deciding on priorities can be confusing and difficult. Some people manage to seize the opportunity to do things they have been putting off; AIDS makes the here and now much more important.

Many have found that the most effective formula is to live 'one day at a time'. This fits in with the unpredictability of the illness and helps focus on 'now', rather than on some vague and indeterminate time in the future.

Living with AIDS often means re-training. It means thinking more of the quality of life than the quantity. People who cope best seem to be those who plan changes in an active and positive way. For example, some people increase the amount of time they spend socially – with partners, family and friends, especially in talking and relaxing, which is important in maintaining good communication and mutual trust. Some people take the opportunity to develop entirely new interests.

Manage energy

Energy levels can often be unpredictable and some people get upset when they find they cannot do everything they want to. Weeks in which it has been possible to live normally can be followed by periods of feeling totally drained. There may be times when someone may have to spend the day in bed, or have a rest in the afternoon. It is important to rest when necessary, but it is not always easy to accept the need to do so.

Anyone who is feeling exhausted a lot of the time because he or she is doing too much needs to take a careful look at his or her activities to see if they are all really necessary. Conversely, people who spend a lot of time in bed unnecessarily may be avoiding confronting something. A counsellor may be able to help if this is a particular problem. The key is to set realistic goals and plan achievable activities.

Keep up interests

Keeping up interests is important in its own right. It is important to avoid becoming submerged by AIDS. Keeping a healthy interest in things is likely to contribute to staying healthy. Keeping busy can mean life continues much as normal, bringing with it interests and maintaining normal social contacts.

It is easy for people with AIDS to isolate themselves and then begin to think that nobody cares and eventually become cut off altogether. Withdrawal is something to be aware of and fight against – perhaps by sticking to a schedule of keeping in contact with people, going out and sharing activities once more. Some people begin to interest themselves in new activities and meet a new set of people. Another source of support may be self-help groups of people in similar situations – see page 59.

Get support

Support from others is really important. No one should hesitate to ask for it; people are often too shy or too uneasy to offer it themselves. In different ways partners, family and friends can make it possible for someone to remain independent. Not only can they help in practical ways but they can listen, hold, laugh and cry. They can also help cushion someone from the 'downs' as well as celebrate the 'ups'. Some people with AIDS have been loath to ask for help because they have become convinced that they cannot give anything back. Yet those who have just taken the time to say how much particular friends or carers have meant have found that this is all that was needed.

Control anxiety

No one with HIV can avoid anxiety. David Miller in *Living with Aids and HIV* (see page 289) describes some different concerns voiced by people with HIV and

AIDS. Apart from fears about the short- and long-term outcome of the infection, they included worries about hostility and rejection, the ability of family and friends to cope, loss of privacy, loss of independence and fears of isolation.

Anxiety and stress can have physical symptoms as well as emotional and psychological ones, and it is important that these are controlled. A starting point may be to decide to face the situation head on, and see it as an opportunity for taking charge. Some people find it helpful to identify each worry and work out ways of combating each one separately. This may involve learning to think more positively about the situation or about oneself, or adopting a specific plan of action. Some people find it useful to write their plans down, along with a list of the strengths and pluses they will bring to the situation. It may help to give each activity an enjoyment rating. It may also be useful to list negative thoughts and discuss them. Some can even be put to the test – people who think their friends would no longer want to see them can usually be proved wrong, for example.

Depression is totally understandable to begin with, but it usually lifts after a time. If it persists in a severe form it may be necessary to take deliberate steps to stop being drawn into a downward spiral. Talking to someone about these concerns is likely to be extremely helpful. More information about counselling and sources of help is given in Chapter 4.

It is important to learn to relax. Brief details of organisations which may be of interest appear on page 273. Various complementary therapies involve relaxation; see page 200 for how to find a practitioner.

Think about diet and exercise

A healthy diet and adequate exercise are important elements in staying healthy. It is essential not to make too many dramatic changes all at once as these may be difficult to cope with. Too much exercise can be a hazard in itself and trying to give up cigarettes or alcohol suddenly can be stressful.

Talk about feelings

Many people find it very difficult to talk honestly about what they feel. It is even less easy for people with AIDS because their preoccupations are often about difficult issues such as loss, anger, death, sex and disability. Strong feelings of loss and grief can be overwhelming, and can lead to severe depression, withdrawal and isolation. Bottling up feelings takes energy which could be better used fighting back. The more a person with AIDS is able to talk and to seek support the easier communication becomes.

Counsellors

Talking to an experienced counsellor can help someone find ways of coping with the situation in a constructive way. Someone who is detached may be able to give a fresh perspective and suggest ways of dealing with things which hadn't been thought of. Talking about feelings, even if it doesn't change the facts of the situation, can reduce negative feelings of anger, loss, depression or helplessness.

Many individuals and organisations provide a way of talking about these feelings and are expert enough to help break through the barriers that lie in the way. They include telephone helplines, support groups, counsellors, social workers, health advisors, friends and clergy. Particularly important are the self-help groups who can draw on first-hand experience. Details of these are to be found throughout this book. What is offered will vary from place to place, but it should be possible to find someone who can offer a safe and supportive environment in which to talk in tranquillity and confidence. Many people find that they begin to meet new people as they attend support groups and find that their circle of supporters grows accordingly.

Talking to a partner

Some couples have found that coming to terms with HIV has provided an opportunity to enrich their relationship. Taking stock of the present and planning the future seems to help both become closer and more mutually supportive.

About carers

Who should care?

When it comes to caring, there is no set pattern, nor is one type of arrangement necessarily better than another. Some people are supported by a partner as part of a very close relationship. Others choose to manage for themselves with occasional help from friends or family. Sometimes groups of friends co-operate with one another to provide whatever is needed at the time.

It is natural for partners, close relatives and very good friends to become carers automatically. Other people may be asked to help or may be thinking about what they could offer. If you are in this position you should consider things very carefully first. You also need to be aware of your own motives and attitudes. People who offer help just because they feel they ought to carry out 'good works' are unlikely to make good carers. Some people are drawn towards caring because they want to feel wanted and necessary. Caring may give some people a role in life or a special identity. Some even see some kind of glamour in caring for someone with AIDS, particularly while it is so much in the news.

The carer should ask himself whether he's fulfilling the needs of the person with AIDS or just his own needs

This is not to say you shouldn't have any needs which are met by being a carer. But they should not be your prime motivation, or get in the way of giving appropriate care.

Sometimes people are very concerned and offer help to satisfy their own needs, but don't have any real commitment. Carers sometimes feel a greater understanding and commitment is going to develop than actually does; sometimes they are looking for some emotional benefit themselves; this can be a dangerous expectation

Some people have a natural aptitude for caring for the sick. For others the practicalities of nursing or the helplessness of an ill person are daunting, and it is unlikely that they will make good carers. You should try to match the care you can offer to the skills (and time) that you have.

I expected three hours of domestic work two days a week on a flexible basis. It turned out to be two very full days. I suddenly began to have my own personal problems and I began to resent being asked to do more and more each week

Caring for someone with AIDS may be a somewhat open-ended commitment, and you have to be sure you will be able to continue to give the help you promise.

Commitment and continuity are most important. The person with AIDS needs to feel he or she can rely on you and that you won't let him or her down – they need to feel safe

Some friends are a burden, they don't help – they promise things then they don't carry it through. Stick to your word, it's vital

It goes without saying that if you find you are making judgements about the lifestyle of the person with AIDS or the way in which he or she became infected with HIV, you are not the right person to help.

Finally you should appreciate that the relationship between a carer and a person with HIV is usually an immensely important one. It is important that you do not end up acting artificially. If you don't say what you feel or don't behave honestly you are likely to undermine the relationship.

Be honest with yourself and honest with the person you are supporting. Don't go in with any false pretensions or promise the world. You may be the only person they have any contact with as everyone else has left. So you're their only link – be very, very honest

Dealing with differences of view is sometimes difficult. One carer found he was helping someone who was violently racist and took issue with this; much argument followed. As a carer you don't have to suppress your own opinions and ideas because you are working with someone who is ill. Cosseting someone can be patronising, but how far you go is a matter for your own judgement.

Sometimes the problem is a conflict of personality and sometimes just differences in belief and outlook. Some carers have become so exasperated by unpredictable behaviour that they have given up. If you have any of these difficulties and feel that they cannot be resolved you may be able to help find someone else to take over, if you are not the only potential carer.

What should carers do?

Again, there are no rules. How much and what you will do will depend on what the person with AIDS wants, your relationship, what you are *able* to do and so on. All this will have to be worked out individually.

Guidance is given in the various chapters of this book on various issues which cause common problems. Although this book is dedicated to carers, this does not imply that it is necessarily the carer who should take the initiative, find out information or make arrangements. Who does what will depend on the wishes of the person with AIDS and on whatever is appropriate at the time.

Sometimes friends who are less immediately involved are at a loss when thinking about what they can do or even about how to behave. The following ideas have been adapted from the *National AIDS Manual* (described on page 56):

- Don't avoid your friend. Be the friend you've always been, especially now when it's most important
- Touch your friend. A simple squeeze or a hug or a kiss can show that you care
- Phone up and ask if it's all right to come and visit. Don't be offended if it's not – it could just be too tiring to see anyone that day
- Don't keep a stiff upper lip – respond to emotions. Weep or laugh naturally – it's a great relief to share strong feelings
- Have a meal together. Offer to cook. Or ring up and suggest bringing round a favourite dish. Or invite your friend out to a restaurant
- Go for a walk or outing, but check that the person you are with is not overdoing it
- Offer to help with any letters, forms or bureaucracy that could be difficult or tiring
- Help do the shopping
- Organise a rota of friends to help with practical chores around the house: cooking, shopping, cleaning
- Go on holiday or for a short break together. Offer to decorate a room at home or bring flowers to cheer up a hospital room
- Check to see if your friend's partner, flatmate or carer needs a break from time to time. They may need someone to talk to as well
- Bring books, magazines, tapes, records, posters or anything else that might be welcomed
- Don't be afraid to ask about illness, or about how your friend is feeling. Don't pursue it if your friend doesn't want to talk about it and don't overdo it
- You don't always have to talk. Much can be expressed just by being together, listening to music, watching TV, holding hands
- Tell your friend they're looking good when they are
- Encourage your friend to make decisions and keep control
- If you say you'll do something make sure you do it
- Gossip can be healthy. Keep your friend up to date on mutual friends and other common interests, current events, the news and so on
- Send a card to say hello from time to time

- You can make suggestions but don't lecture or get angry at your friend if he or she seems to be handling any illness in a way you think is wrong. You may not understand what the feelings are and why certain choices are being made
- Bring a positive attitude. Talk about the future. Treatments for opportunistic infections are much more effective than they used to be. There's a lot of room for hope. Belief in the future and hope may well be crucial therapies till the time when AIDS may no longer be life-threatening

Some key points

After diagnosis

Reactions to being diagnosed as HIV-positive and as having ARC or AIDS can be similar. The following may apply in either situation. There is no one predictable reaction. For some people, their diagnosis comes as a complete shock. For others, it's almost a relief to have a suspicion confirmed. However, the period following the news can be extremely traumatic. For many people, the emotional effects of the diagnosis are much more severe than any physical signs of it. Partners and close friends may share the trauma.

> *It's like a nightmare. You keep expecting the phone to ring and be told it's all a mistake. But the phone doesn't ring and it's true*

There is little a book can do to guide you or the person with HIV through the days which follow. You will need to rely on your own sensitivity, your understanding and on the bond between you.

Shock, anger, fear, numbness and plain disbelief are all common first reactions, and are to be expected. Individual reactions will depend to some extent on personality, the way people approach problems generally, the support and care they are given by others and on the circumstances at the time of diagnosis. Some people become 'more like themselves' while others may behave in a way which is out of character, which makes it all the harder to know what to do. Some people are already ill at the time of diagnosis and don't really have a chance to come to terms with it at all.

Some may deny or ignore the diagnosis altogether. This is a natural way of cushioning the jolt of the news and the enormous implications it may have. As time goes on most people feel more able to talk more about their feelings and what they want to do. If denial persists it can cause great problems because the person who has been diagnosed may not have the opportunity to adjust and may not take steps to stay healthy. This attitude will not help anyone to stay in control of the situation and you as a carer may need to make sure it is discussed honestly. Body Positive (page 59) may be able to help.

Some people can break down altogether with frequent bouts of sobbing and emotional outbursts. Others withdraw physically or emotionally after the diagnosis. They can become very unresponsive and don't seem to take anything in. With so much to deal with they may need periods alone until they feel more able to communicate. Don't be offended by this. You need to be aware of the fine distinction between solitude and loneliness. People with AIDS have sometimes become lonely because companions have disappeared after their first offers of help and support have been turned down. You have to judge how best to remain in the background while being able to offer support when it is wanted. You need to let them know you are there without being intrusive. Never force contact without very good reason, such as a real worry about someone's emotional balance. It is sometimes very difficult to sort out the difference between the needs of the person you are caring for and a need to show your own care and concern.

Anger is a common emotion, and is usually a healthy reaction. It becomes dangerous only when someone is unable to express it in a constructive way or suppresses it entirely. Sometimes anger may be misdirected – to you as the carer, to a partner, doctor or even society in general. If it is directed inwards it can lead to feelings of guilt or to an extremely destructive process of self-denigration. When someone is unable to express anger, pent-up feelings may explode in outbursts over minor occurrences, such as a row about whose turn it is to do the washing-up. Try not to over-react to these flare-ups, but use the opportunity to talk through the situation as calmly as you can.

Periods of depression are likely to occur regularly. They can sometimes be reduced by talking and by demonstrations of solid support. However, you may find that all your attempts to help don't work, and that everything you do appears to be awkward or wrong. Keep in mind that it is normal to have any of the reactions described. Try not to over-react to changed behaviour or any anger or aggression which seems to be directed at you. You do need to show that you care and that you are *there*. Touch – hugs, kissing, holding hands – is extremely important, not only to show how you feel, but to demonstrate that the diagnosis does not mean that people will keep their distance.

One good way to come to terms with the situation is to make sure you both have full and accurate information. If you are caring for a partner, or are close enough, it is helpful if you both visit a doctor or advisory centre together. Often when people are given a positive diagnosis their minds begin to race and what is said becomes a blur. Much of the counselling and advice given at this time is easily forgotten and may need to be repeated. If there are two of you, it is easier to get things clear.

Don't hesitate to ask questions. Try to pinpoint someone who will be able to answer them later too. It may help to arrange for another appointment just to discuss things more fully. It may also help to work out questions in advance, and have a list to make sure that they are all asked. Many people have found that getting a full explanation has been difficult or that they have been treated unsympathetically. Hospital staff may be short of time (or even of information), or may explain things using medical terms which are unclear or sound menacing.

A good clinic will give clear information, proper counselling and make arrangements for follow-up care. If the clinic is not helpful it is worth one of you checking to see if there is a better one within reach. STD (sexually transmitted disease) or HIV clinics are likely to have the most experience. Your local AIDS helpline (see page 295) or the National AIDS Helpline (see page 56) should be able to tell you what is available where. Local helplines will also know about other local services and may have other useful information, too. It will help both of you to talk to others who are in similar situations, who will be able to reassure and advise.

I get help from my support group at any time; it's very important to be able to share my own distress and get practical back-up

In particular support groups run by people who are HIV-positive themselves, or who have ARC or AIDS, are able to demonstrate how they have found successful ways of living with AIDS:

Body Positive – see page 59

Support groups organised by Terrence Higgins Trust – see page 57

Frontliners – see page 60

Positive Partners – see page 61

Positively Women – see page 221

Also ask your local AIDS helpline or the National AIDS Helpline for information about other centres or organisations.

Being HIV-positive does not mean that the person has AIDS – see page 17. Many people with HIV infection have been fit and well for a number of years. The history of the condition is too short for much to be known about the long term, but many people believe that it is possible to stay healthy for a very long time. Taking positive steps to keep healthy, which may involve sensible eating, exercise, finding appropriate therapies as well as positive thinking are extremely worthwhile. The organisations listed above should be able to advise.

Telling people

Deciding whether to tell anyone is a decision which has to be made by the person with HIV. In times of stress and need most people look to their friends and family for support. One of the ironies about HIV is that at the time of greatest need, many people feel unable to be open. Some are afraid of unleashing discrimination or hostility. For some there is a fear that talking about HIV will reveal more about their sexuality or life-style than they want to share.

It is not easy to predict how people will react when they are told. One person in our survey was 'hurt beyond words' when a friend of fifty years' standing did not make any attempt at all to visit or get in touch after he had been told of the diagnosis. Yet other people have received understanding support from unexpected directions – neighbours who made a point of taking on regular practical tasks; families who came together to support them through thick and thin.

Main partners

Most people will want to tell their current sexual partner. There are many reasons why they should. However, there may be circumstances in which breaking the news can be particularly difficult – for instance bisexual men may not want to broach the subject with their wives. Some people do not want to admit to affairs outside their central relationship because of feelings of shame and guilt, and many people will have a fear of being rejected. But what must be considered are the consequences of not telling.

Careful counselling may be useful and it may be particularly helpful to talk to other people who have faced the same situation – see page 59 for details of Body Positive groups and page 60 for information about Frontliners. The following list of points for a person with HIV to think about has been adapted from the *National AIDS Manual*:

- How much does the partner or lover know about AIDS and HIV infection?
- What is his or her attitude to health generally?
- What is the likely reaction to the news – would he or she just panic, or react positively?
- Would *not* telling put anyone else at risk? If not, what would be achieved by telling?
- How would telling affect the relationship? If you don't tell, what would happen if they were to discover later on?
- Would you be able to keep such an important matter a secret?

Other sexual partners

There may be practical difficulties in tracking down past sexual partners. And it can be difficult to know for how long one has been infectious. People with HIV should tell new partners unless they are absolutely confident of acting in a way which poses no risk.

Family

Some people have the hardest time dealing with their immediate family, particularly if this means telling them they are gay. Worries about how parents may react may be worse if the parents are elderly. It may even be feared that the news could make them ill. If contact with parents has been lost, it can be even more difficult to tell them.

Yet many people have found that families were surprisingly able to accept and cope with the news and were able to offer care and emotional support that could not have been matched by anyone else. Some people have become close to their families for the first time because of AIDS. One mother described how she took the initiative when her son was unable to talk easily about his illness:

> *I phoned him. I was very nervous, it was very difficult. I told him I'd been thinking about it and had to talk to him as my knowledge of the symptoms was that it was only serious if the immune system was breaking down. After a pause, in a very quiet voice, he said: 'yes, that's it exactly'. He was very relieved. I told him: 'You can rely on us, we'll look after you.' I got my husband to phone him and confirm the support*

Even when people cannot face the situation directly they may find a way of dealing with it. One carer described how he had to meet his partner's father 'off the bus from the North'. The father did not know that his son was gay or that he had AIDS; only that he was dying. The son's partner spent a lot of time with him, sharing his grief, hugging, listening and talking through the distressing times which followed. The father at no time acknowledged the relationship between his son and his partner 'almost as if by not doing so he didn't have to deal with it'. This didn't stop him accepting and valuing the support given to him, or affect the support he was able to give to his son.

Owing to fears about the reaction, some parents have been told only towards the terminal stage of an illness. This means that there is little time to adjust, make contact and perhaps heal old wounds. Because the situation is confused by grief, they may be unable to say all the things they would wish to or demonstrate their real feelings. Neither do they have time to learn about the illness and may come to it with all kinds of damaging prejudices. One mother told us that if she had been told sooner she could have helped her son more 'and been more to him'. Some people are deeply hurt because they have not been trusted and have been excluded from the scene. Families who have not been told until after a death are likely to be particularly upset.

Not telling can also be a source of additional worry and stress. Some family members can be more difficult to tell than others. It may be possible to ask a relative who does know to broach the subject with others.

There can be difficulty at keeping up the pretence. One carer described to us how he had to pretend to be a voluntary home-help when a mother visited a son whom she thought had cancer.

Friends

Some people with HIV will not want to hide things from close friends. It is impossible to build up a network of support unless people are told. However, they may hesitate to tell some friends until they are sure that they will react well and will respect the confidence.

Other people

Again, the decision of whom to tell beyond family and friends is one the person with HIV must make. As a rule it is probably best to tell as few people as possible. There are good practical reasons for this. Some people have been dismissed after an employer has been told about the diagnosis. Landlords and even neighbours can make life difficult, too.

It's not always possible to limit the spread of gossip. Hostility and rejection (and the self-conscious attentions of 'do-gooders') can be devastating. Careful thought about who can be trusted to respect the confidence is needed. Thought needs to be given to possible reactions and how they would have to be dealt with. It is always possible to tell people later – but they cannot be *un*told.

Medical and nursing staff (including dentists) are supposed to protect themselves against the possibility of infection as a matter of course. It should not be necessary to tell them anything but people who are HIV-positive may consider it right to do so where contact with blood is possible, for example if surgery is needed.

Dentists should already follow clear guidelines issued by the British Dental Association. However, it may be necessary to check that they are following these guidelines. One guarded way of doing this is for the person with HIV to ask what precautions they take to protect patients from infection. If the answer is unsatisfactory it may be worth changing dentists. The local AIDS helpline or HIV clinic may know of a sympathetic, informed dentist.

Practical matters

There is no simple answer to the question 'How do you care for someone who has AIDS?'. The answers are as different as the people involved. The main aim is to meet the needs of the person you are caring for. As there is no right or wrong way to cope with AIDS, there are no fixed rules for carers to follow.

Three basic starting points are practical help, giving support and taking care of yourself. Some practical tasks and ways of showing support are outlined below with cross-references to information in other chapters. See chapter 19 for information on how to look after yourself. If you want to take things further – for

Practical help

example, by campaigning or contributing to the work of voluntary organisations – see pages 73–81.

Everyday practical tasks may become extremely difficult at times for a person with AIDS. The physical, financial and emotional consequences of the illness can make day-to-day living very complicated. Sorting out practical difficulties may be an area where carers can provide an immense amount of help. But don't just assume responsibility, you must be sure that you are not being domineering. It's too easy to take over and deny someone the right to manage independently. You should aim to help when it is needed and welcome.

Some of the things you may have to help with are described below.

Housing
Having a good standard of accommodation and enough money to pay for heat and light are obvious needs. Without suitable accommodation it is much harder to stay healthy and very poor housing can be downright dangerous. Yet many people with AIDS have difficulties with accommodation. Dealing with the legal side of housing problems, with the various organisations concerned with housing, claiming welfare benefits and finding suitable accommodation can all be unpleasant and traumatic. Chapter 7 gives details of what accommodation may be available for people who are homeless and an outline of some legal considerations for tenants and home owners. Chapter 9 gives details of financial help available towards housing costs.

Financial problems
Many people with AIDS are unable to work and face increased expenses such as special diets and the cost of being ill. Carers may have to leave work or take unpaid leave, and may also have to find extra money. Details of the main welfare benefits, and how to claim them, are given on pages 143–75. Information on charities which give money to individuals is given on pages 176–83.

Legal questions
A summary of common legal issues, such as your rights under employment law if you are ill or caring for someone who is ill, power of attorney and wills, are discussed in Chapter 5. Information on how to get free legal advice is on page 103.

Transport

Many more people with AIDS are being treated as outpatients nowadays. Transport to and from hospital and for social and other purposes can be in short supply. Some are unable to drive and may be unable or unwilling to use public transport. Details of Dial-a-Ride, special taxi schemes and transport services run by volunteers are outlined on pages 138–9. On page 153 information on discounted fares and concessionary parking is given.

Nursing

Carers may need to provide basic nursing. Practical guidance is given in chapter 6. Details of domiciliary support and nursing help on page 50.

Domestic tasks

Everyday practical tasks – shopping, cooking, cleaning, laundry and so on – can take an enormous amount of time and energy. Some people with AIDS will want to continue to do these things for themselves for as long as possible; others will be only too happy to abdicate responsibility. Some carers may prefer to take on these tasks personally. But various sorts of help are available, including Home-Helps (see page 54), Meals on Wheels (page 55), and other volunteers (page 74). Laundry can be a special problem if someone becomes incontinent or needs many changes of bedclothes – see page 37.

Round-the-clock care

There may be times when a carer needs to be within reach 24 hours a day. It is inadvisable and impractical to try to do this single-handed. However, it is often difficult to get outside help, particularly during the daytime and after midnight – details on page 63.

Taking a break

An important duty is to take care of yourself. If you're exhausted, bad-tempered or just at the end of your tether you won't be able to give the kind of care that you would wish to. The importance of taking a break cannot be overstressed. There are various ways of doing this and several organisations which can help. Information starts on page 277.

Giving support

It's worth remembering that by definition a support is just something that is there – a crutch, a prop, a pillar: something doing very little itself beyond being in the right place and being strong enough to stop something else falling down.

Just being there when wanted is a very important part of the support that friends or family can provide.

Being there

Being there is your first and main role. This means not only being physically there when you are needed but also paying full attention – surprisingly rare in practice. It doesn't mean being around all the time. There are likely to be times when you are not wanted and you should not be offended by this.

When someone is ill old friends can disappear, usually because they don't know what to say or how to behave in the circumstances. If you are closer than this, you may be able to encourage others to visit and help them get over any awkwardness. Your own sense of ease will help. A group of friends who visit may reduce any concern that particular friends are being imposed upon. Some people with AIDS worry about this and it can be hard to convince them that friends wouldn't be there if they didn't want to be.

Being there may mean:

- Spending time together just to relax. If you spend time together only when you are exhausted or in a rush, you will have no opportunity and probably no wish to discuss problems or worries. If you are the main carer this may mean relying on others to take over some time-consuming tasks. You may have to spend money or make the effort to ask for help, but it's usually worth it.
- Planning your time together so it's spent in as enjoyable a way as possible. This helps to turn your minds to the positive side of living. Don't be afraid of humour or sharing the funny side of things.
- Remembering to pass on good feelings – it is much easier to talk if you are both sure of the relationship. Don't forget the importance of touch.
- Trying not to bottle up anxieties. Talk about your concerns.
- Getting outside advice or counselling, if appropriate – see page 83.

I could have done with some professional advice some weeks ago. It might have saved our relationship – but it seems too late now. I wanted to talk to someone outside our relationship, totally detached

Listening and talking
Listening and talking may be the most valuable things you can do. Sometimes the

person with AIDS may want to talk and at other times may just want to sit in silence; this does not mean that your presence is any less important.

Listening and talking are skills that take practice to perfect. It's all too easy to interpret rather than listen. Some people unconsciously translate what is being expressed into their own words, and in doing so change the meaning, which can lead to a total misunderstanding. A few examples of common problems are:

Hearing only what you want to hear – it is easy to listen selectively, and shut out anything that feels uncomfortable or is difficult to deal with. This may be done by saying: 'I don't want to talk about that now', by just ignoring what has been said or even actually not hearing it. Probably the more you are able to deal with issues that make you feel uncomfortable the better.

Replaying old tunes – instead of hearing what is being said it is easy to hear the echoes of a situation from the past, and react to that instead.

Not taking the time to listen – it's possible to be irritated when your attention is demanded when you're busy or just about to go out. Or you're feeling hurt because he or she didn't listen to you when you needed to talk.

Hidden meanings – people quite often find difficulty in saying what the problem really is: for example, claiming 'I'm all right' when there is clearly something wrong. You will need to be alert to coded messages and follow them up.

You may have to develop your own ways of finding out what the trouble is. One way is to start asking general questions – about the day, TV programmes and 'gossipy stuff' – until talking becomes easier.

> *I just wait for him to tell me . . . I could coax things, but if you're in a bad mood, you don't want to be forced, do you?*

Don't be scared of discussing the illness, the future or whatever, honestly and directly. Be easy to talk to. But don't force conversation on to topics the person doesn't want to discuss.

You may find worries about very basic matters, for which great reassurance is needed. Try your utmost to stop the person feeling guilt or blame.

Help people to come to terms with societal attitudes, oppression from childhood, . . . feelings of worthlessness, hopelessness; gay people have this reinforced – 'I deserve to die'

Coping with changes

Each day is likely to be different. Energy levels can change from day to day or even from hour to hour. You may find that the person has moods which are extremely changeable, moving from calmness into a temper tantrum, rages or bouts of tears in minutes. In some circumstances people can be hyper-sensitive to extremely small things – nuances of words, tone of voice and so on. Sometimes people rage against the person they are closest to, who are unable and unwilling to retreat from the situation. Some of the things said to you may be extremely hurtful. 'The only thing to do may be to put up your armour and not take it personally; you can be very hurt otherwise', as one advised. It may help to remember that outbursts directed at you may really be a sign of your closeness and that you are trusted. Try to remain constant so you will become a stable point to focus on.

His state of mind is deteriorating, getting more irritable and depressed. The way he treats me is getting worse – either he is very very affectionate or he says things which he knows will hurt me.

I've never experienced such anger – he'd scream, then burst into tears, then would say: 'Don't touch me!'

These reactions are totally understandable – there may be uncertainty about the future, a feeling of injustice or a feeling of being powerless, for example. There may be other causes too:

- Drugs – mood changes are an unfortunate side effect of some medications.
- Illness – even when there are no drugs involved, the body undergoes a number of changes during serious illness which can affect moods.
- Fatigue.
- HIV in the brain – changes in personality can occur as a direct result of HIV acting on the central nervous system and on the brain. Symptoms can include a tendency to become more withdrawn and less lively. Some people find it difficult to concentrate and have problems with memory – such as being able to find the right word, for example. Occasionally they have difficulty doing small practical things: fumbling, for instance, with buttons.

Do your best to ignore the bad moods. Even when this is a strain, try to maintain your sense of humour. Sometimes anger can turn to laughter if you can point out the funny side of a situation. Don't be afraid to tell anyone else who is helping with the caring about any difficulties, so that they do not over-react.

Dealing with stress and depression

Stress and depression are experienced by everybody at some time. It would be extremely odd if someone with AIDS did not go through periods of great strain; sometimes this will be almost unbearable. But even when there seem to be valid reasons for them, *prolonged* periods of stress or depression are not a good sign and may contribute to a breakdown in health. Stress cannot necessarily be eliminated but it can be recognised, controlled and contained.

Counselling (see page 83) and contact with self-help groups (see chapter 3) are likely to help. In some cases a doctor may help.

You should try to make it easy for the person you are caring for to express the fears and anxieties he or she may be experiencing. If you are a close friend or a trusted acquaintance he or she may be able to confess and acknowledge deep-rooted feelings. These may be long-concealed doubts, terror or just awful uncertainty. Being able to share them may greatly reduce anxiety. The person with AIDS should feel free to express all this without inhibition; don't be put off by crying, incoherence or any other signs of deep emotion. Try to make it obvious that you will do everything you can to help.

It may help to list the causes of stress (some of them may be quite simple practical problems) so that a plan of action can be agreed for each. Some people compile lists with a timetable, and note the results of any steps taken. This is encouraging evidence that problems are being faced and *controlled*. It also makes it more difficult to ignore some of the causes of stress.

On page 272 we describe some methods of relaxation and sources of relaxation exercises; see also page 200 for where to go for information about complementary therapies.

Coping with dementia

Dementia affects only a minority of people with HIV; some people may have minor problems with memory and slower reactions for other reasons. Dementia affects people in different ways, and to different extents. It can be distressing, particularly when it appears in someone who is young. However, mild difficulties with speech and movement need not cause too many problems. It is better to admit to any problems that do exist than try to pretend they are not there.

One particular problem is forgetfulness. People with dementia often don't remember to keep appointments, they may forget to take their drugs or even forget to eat. Because they can forget what they have just said they tend to repeat themselves endlessly, and this can make communication difficult and tiring. Dementia does not usually mean a person is totally incapable.

> *. . . asked me to do shopping for him. He'd also asked somebody else. I made a joke about the two lots of shopping and having driven for an hour across London*

> *He never got confused over his pills, but he wouldn't take them. I found them behind his teeth or under the bedclothes*

One carer described how the person he was caring for was totally disoriented about time and couldn't remember recent events ('I was forever starting to read *The Wind in the Willows* again!'), but he enjoyed watching quiz programmes and would get all the answers right.

Lots of attention may be needed at this time, particularly when someone lives alone. Try to do what seems appropriate. It may be better just to listen to music together at times when conversation is too difficult, for example. A big problem is the availability of carers during the day when people are at work. You may be able to get help from a voluntary organisation or from the NHS – see chapter 19.

AVERT have a free leaflet on Dementia – see page 222 for address.

Worries about appearance

People with AIDS often worry about the way they look, sometimes even when they look well and attractive. Losing weight is of great concern because it is one of the symptoms of AIDS, and is often thought to be an indicator of health. Other causes of distress are changes to the texture of hair, hair loss and skin problems. Whatever the cause, you may need to give reassurance about appearance.

> *People need to be prepared for what they face. I was shocked at his appearance first . . . I was ashamed at my shock; five minutes and I was over it. It was difficult not to feel bad*

Kaposi's sarcoma, because it is so visible and can appear so extensively, can be very distressing:

> *X became depressed at speed of KS lesions over face and body. Had two very bad reactions to chemotherapy – face swollen and was really upset by that. Didn't want to be seen or go out*

Although there is an understandable tendency for carers and visitors to pretend nothing has changed this may not be helpful in the long run. One carer approached the subject directly by saying: 'God, what has happened to your face?' and found that this made it possible to talk freely.

KS lesions on parts of the body which show can be disguised cosmetically; the Red Cross will visit to show how this is done – see page 75 for details.

If you can you should discourage an obsessional interest in the way someone's body may be changing. This is an understandable symptom of anxiety. For example some people develop a habit of searching their bodies for KS lesions which can become so ingrained that it stops them going out. Try to persuade them to stop. If they are not aware that this kind of obsession is irrational, you may need to seek professional psychiatric help.

Let's Face It

Let's Face It is an organisation which exists to provide counselling and mutual support for people who look 'different'. Although not set up for people with AIDS, many of their members have been affected by illnesses which has affected their appearance. They hold regular meetings, usually in hospitals in fifteen centres in England and Scotland but the network is expanding into other areas.

> Let's Face It
> 10 Wood End
> Crowthorne
> Berkshire RG11 6DQ   (0344) 774405

Tips from Let's Face It to help people talking to someone who is worried about their appearance:

- look them in the eyes
- accept their feelings

44

- acknowledge their anger, fear and bewilderment . . . and perhaps your own
- remember that laughter is often the best medicine
- if you love them, tell them so

Coping with physical weakness

Some people become completely dependent on their carers at times, and are unable to move independently.

> *In the last four weeks he never slept. For a month I sat with him and never slept in my bed*

The section on nursing describes some of the tasks you may have to do, and a district nurse (page 50) should be able to arrange practical assistance and show you how best to help.

Difficult situations

Some situations have proved to be particularly difficult for carers. One is the problem of being overwhelmed. For example, if someone starts to have episodes of illness or gives up a job and so spends most time at home, the carer can suddenly find that he or she is also spending all his time at home, and can become desperate with a sense of unrelieved responsibility. This situation can be avoided only by recognising it early on, talking about it and enlisting help from others.

> *I feel all the pressure and responsibility is on me and he plays on my emotions. I feel mentally drained and wish I had never got this far*

It is important to remember that people who are ill do not necessarily become saints. People who were demanding or sometimes unreasonable before the diagnosis may become more so afterwards. You will have to judge how far you are willing to make allowances for the illness. Honesty seems to work best:

> *. . . always on the phone – taking advantage of my goodwill and expecting me to ferry him around . . . I eventually had to state the limits; he understood and accepted*

> *You have to be very assertive, especially when someone is so manipulative. He knew how to keep me there an extra few hours. It was difficult to say no and I gave in. I should have set limits – there was no reason why he shouldn't have been alone for four or five hours*

Significant dates can be difficult – the anniversary of the diagnosis, the date given in a prognosis and celebrations such as birthdays, holidays, Christmas and Easter. These events can take on a morbid importance – 'Will this be my last birthday?'

If you are aware of these likely crunch points in advance it is possible to lessen the emotional impact they may have. One way of doing this is to devise different ways of spending days which look like being difficult – for example, arrange for the day to be filled with events and happenings, perhaps as a surprise. A trip out, visits by friends or an unexpected party are possibilities. Christmas can perhaps be dealt with by deciding not to celebrate it in a traditional way, but by going somewhere which does not have previous associations.

Stigma

You may meet ignorance and prejudice. If you come across these attitudes, you may choose to argue or ignore them. However, part of your job may be to screen the person with AIDS from people who are likely to react badly.

Real prejudice is hard to dislodge, and you may feel that this is not the time to try. However, many people's prejudices fade in the light of accurate information. It may be worthwhile explaining about AIDS, about ways HIV is transmitted or about anything else which is causing difficulties. Sometimes people can be converted to your side in the most spectacular manner.

Some guidance for people who have difficulty adjusting to the fact that a relative or close friend is gay is given on page 209.

Fear of a bad reaction or of the news of the diagnosis has sometimes stopped people seeking help. It is worth taking cautious soundings before writing off a source of help. Local Aidslines should know which services you can use without worry and those which are best avoided.

Dealing with obsessions

Some people develop obsessional thoughts. These may disappear naturally in time but if they don't can become a major problem. They can sometimes be difficult to treat.

People with AIDS may have obsessions about things outside the illness, about AIDS itself and about related matters such as irrational and unfounded fears about who they might have infected in the past. Some people over-react to slight or imagined symptoms.

A starting point is to discuss any obsessional thoughts with the person and try to sort out the basic worries which may lie beneath them. Sometimes the root cause is depression, and treatment may be needed for this. The first step is for the person to recognise that certain patterns of thoughts are irrational. After this he or she may be able to get into the habit of deliberately thinking of something else or doing something sufficiently absorbing when these thoughts occur. It is easier to become obsessive when the mind is unoccupied, so keeping busy may help.

Counselling or professional help may be needed. A doctor or hospital consultant should be able to give reassurance that concerns about minor symptoms are not the signs of a new infection or the beginning of a decline into further illness.

Facing death

At times both you and the person you are caring for will inevitably think about death. Whether you choose to voice these thoughts – and how – will depend on you and your relationship. But generally, silence is unlikely to bring you any closer. On this subject it is impossible to know without asking how even the person you are closest to feels. And because feelings and thoughts change with time you cannot assume that you can know once and for all. Your own moods, state of health and changing circumstances will also have an effect on you and you may find expressions of your own attitudes to death range from flippancy to tears.

It may be important for both of you to be able to acknowledge the possibility of death and talk about the reality of dying. Any decision not to talk about it should be mutually understood and explicitly agreed – you shouldn't avoid the subject because of a misguided wish to avoid topics which might be upsetting.

For you as the carer the fear is likely to be one of loss and how life is going to be afterwards. This can be made worse when everyday tasks seem difficult, when you are tired and the person you are caring for is unappreciative or irritating.

Some partners talk about plans for the long-term future together. It may help to write down some thoughts you may want to come back to later. This discussion can be painful. But it has the advantage that you are still together at the time. And this sense of togetherness can be preserved beyond the initial shock of death by knowing that you and your partner both planned for the future together.

In chapter 17 grief and bereavement are discussed in more detail.

3

Help, information and services

In this chapter we describe the main services, practical help and support available to people with AIDS and their carers. In some areas there are special teams whose job it is to provide or co-ordinate services but elsewhere the person with AIDS or yourself as carer will have to organise your own network.

Finding out what's available

Services and facilities differ widely from area to area. To make effective use of the help which does exist, you need to find out how the local system works in practice, not just in theory.

Many people have a hard time getting the information they need. There is no magic formula. If you are lucky you will find a helpful and knowledgeable person straight away. If you are not, you will have to dig around. The key to getting the information you need is to keep on asking questions. Surprisingly many people don't volunteer information but will give it willingly enough if asked directly. Apart from all the people and groups described in this chapter, other sources to try locally are:

- Citizens Advice Bureau
- the public library
- the Community Health Council (Local Health Council in Scotland; District Committee in Northern Ireland) which works to improve the services provided by the District Health Authority, and should be well informed about local health services. It will help with complaints about the Health Service, including about doctors
- the Council for Voluntary Service (depending on where you live may be called Voluntary Service Council, Voluntary Action Group or Rural Community Council), which co-ordinates voluntary efforts. Look in the phone book under these names or under Charitable and Benevolent Organisations in the Yellow Pages.

Help through doctors

Records kept by a London home support team showed that in 1987/8 nearly half of their clients with AIDS had no contact with a GP, and of those who were registered over a third hadn't told the doctor about their infection. The main reason for not registering or telling the GP was a fear of lack of confidentiality – sometimes because GPs' records are accessible to anyone working in the surgery. The other main reasons were worries that the doctor would be hostile or have little understanding of the situation. The home support team themselves reported that on one occasion they had had to contact up to 15 surgeries to find a doctor who would take on someone with AIDS.

Some people have never been registered with a doctor and so have not had a chance to build up any kind of relationship with one. Some are treated in hospital from the beginning and have continued to be supervised from hospital.

Yet the family doctor is usually the key to the rest of the Health Service. GPs can arrange for medical or nursing help and will arrange for specialists if necessary. A good doctor will help anyone with HIV to get the best out of the Health Service and will usually be essential if treatment at home is needed or preferred. He or she will help monitor health and work out appropriate treatments. Because a GP is so important it is essential to find one who is sympathetic, knowledgeable and helpful. It is usually a good idea for partners and close friends to talk to doctors too, provided the person with AIDS agrees.

The GP's attitude is probably more important than special knowledge of HIV-related illnesses because many of the opportunistic infections which can develop are the same as, or similar to, other illnesses that GPs deal with. Also, every Health District should have a designated physician with special training in HIV, who has responsibility for keeping up to date with the latest developments and ensuring that information reaches the medical staff who need it. A good GP will keep up with the latest knowledge and take care to obtain any information needed to treat a patient.

Doctors have been given guidelines about confidentiality and HIV – see page 52. *The National AIDS Manual* (see page 56) suggests that anyone particularly concerned about this should ask cautious questions about the kind of details the GP would record on medical notes. Interviews with unsympathetic GPs can then be terminated before any information has been given, and without anything being put on a medical record. A person with HIV may want to change doctors if he or she isn't getting appropriate support or understanding, or if the doctor treats other members of the family.

Anyone is free to choose and change their own doctor. Local NHS GPs are listed in the Family Practitioners Committee Medical List (England and Wales), Primary Care List (Scotland) or the Central Services Agency List (Northern Ireland). These lists can be seen at your local Community Health Council (or Local Health Council in Scotland, District Committee in Northern Ireland), post office, library, police station or Citizens Advice Bureau. This will give basic information such as surgery times and appointment systems. For more information go to the *Medical Directory* (in larger libraries).

Better still is a more personal view from people who have had experience of the doctor. Local support groups, the STD or HIV clinic, or a local AIDS helpline may be able to help. Anyone with HIV should go and see a prospective GP before deciding finally. Note that GPs do not have to take on anybody who asks; some busy doctors close their books.

When someone wants to change doctors, both the old and the new doctor have to sign his or her medical card unless the reason for the change is a change of address. No reasons have to be given for changing doctors, although the new one may well ask why the change is being made. If a patient doesn't want to see the old doctor this can be done by sending a letter and the medical card to the FPC. GPs can arrange for various community services, including those that follow.

Health visitors

Health visitors are nurses who give advice on health and welfare to people in their own homes. They can advise on diet, exercise and the practical problems of being ill at home, including emotional problems. Health visitors know a great deal about local services and can advise on help from the NHS, social services and voluntary organisations.

Some health authorities have a clinical nurse who will counsel and provide support for people who are HIV-positive or who have ARC or AIDS and for their families. They can also liaise with GPs and hospital consultants.

District nurses

District nurses are qualified nurses who have had further training in order to care for people at home. They provide a comprehensive service and will help with nursing tasks such as giving injections, changing dressings, helping with lifting, bathing and so on. They will also teach carers how to do these practical tasks. They also advise on how to cope with problems such as incontinence (see page 117), immobility and bed sores. They sometimes work with *nursing auxiliaries*, who may do some of the basic tasks, and sometimes bathing is carried out by *bathing attendants*. The district nurse may be able to arrange for a night nurse, and for special nursing equipment such as special mattresses (to prevent bed sores) and aids to help with bathing or using the toilet. A district nurse will also liaise with the social services and other organisations if requested to do so.

Anyone not registered with a GP, will find difficulty in getting help from a district nurse because they are all attached to a practice.

Another problem may be the district nurse's uniform. Many people do not want to be visited by people in uniform as this can start neighbours gossiping; in some areas district nurses don't wear them; in others you may be able to persuade them to stop. (See page 51 for information about Macmillan nurses, who carry out related work, but who don't wear uniforms.)

Occupational therapists	Occupational therapists help people manage everyday tasks if these become difficult – see page 54 for a fuller description. OTs based in hospitals work with in-patients and those who have been discharged. Others work from the Social Services department.
Physiotherapists	Physiotherapists work on the body. They help people develop strength, flexibility and movement to enable them to be as independently active as possible. Treatment may be based on exercise, or heat, light or massage or a combination. Some physiotherapists visit, others work in hospitals or rehabilitation centres.
Community psychiatric nurses	These nurses are trained in psychiatry and help people with mental health problems. They can visit at home and give advice, as well as some practical help. They will speak to the GP if a change of treatment is needed. Some may be able to provide counselling or advise where to go to get it. They can be particularly helpful for someone who becomes depressed for long periods, or has special problems overcoming anger or fear.
Nursing or health aids	Equipment such as special mattresses (to minimise pressure sores), incontinence pads and commodes is sometimes provided by the local health authority (and sometimes by health and social services jointly). These items can be obtained through a GP, district nurse, social worker, OT or health visitor.
Making it possible for carers to take a break	In some cases, at certain times – during a bout of illness, say – someone with AIDS may need a great deal of support. Sometimes a carer will need a break, or just some time alone. A GP may be able to help by finding someone to fill in. See pages 280–7 for more information.
Macmillan teams	There are over 200 NHS 'Macmillan' teams (sometimes known as Home Care teams) in the UK. They were originally set up to help people with cancer but will, depending on the policy of the Health District, help people with any incurable disease. They are all experienced senior nurses who are skilled in counselling and able to advise on caring for the patient and on practical and emotional concerns. Macmillan nurses have a lot of experience in helping with the problems of families and carers. They do not wear uniforms. It is up to each Health District to decide on priorities of Macmillan nurses, but their job is primarily to work as part of the home support team and help with pain and symptom control, emotional problems and so on. Doctors, hospital or district nurses will tell you about the

responsibilities of Macmillan nurses in your area. If you have problems get in touch with the co-ordinating organisation:

Cancer Relief (Macmillan Fund)
Anchor House
15-19 Britten Street
London SW3 3TY   01-351 7811

The Macmillan Fund also gives grants to people with cancer – see page 180.

Marie Curie Cancer Care

The Marie Curie Community Nursing Service provides nurses to help nurse people with cancer who are being looked after at home. If the person you are caring for has cancer (Kaposi's sarcoma, for example) this organisation should be able to help. A nurse will assess needs and then decide what can be provided. Marie Curie nurses enable carers to get adequate rest by spending the night or part of the day with patients and by giving all the practical nursing care needed during that time. This service is free; apply to the Community Nursing Officer in your health authority. If you have problems, contact:

Marie Curie Cancer Care
Community Nursing Department
28 Belgrave Square
London SW1X 8QG   01-235 3325

Marie Curie Cancer Care
21 Rutland Street
Edinburgh EH1 2AH   031-229 8332

Obtaining other services

The GP can also be very useful in supporting the case for getting services from your local authority and in obtaining certain welfare benefits.

Confidentiality

All GPs and doctors, and receptionists at surgeries, are bound to keep medical information confidential. Similarly, all nurses, including health visitors and district nurses who visit at home, are obliged to follow the *Code of Professional Conduct for the Nurse*, which requires that information be kept confidential and secure.

Duty of care

All nurses have a duty to take care of all patients, and are professionally obliged to offer appropriate care to those needing it. In the past some health care workers believed that they might be at particular risk in some circumstances – if they were pregnant, for example. It is now known that there are no particular risks of infection from AIDS for health care workers. Refusing to care for any patient is a serious matter and if you come across this it should be reported to the local supervisor or the Director of Nursing Services – your Health Authority will tell you who to contact. Failing this, try the United Kingdom Central Council for Nursing, Midwifery and Health Visiting, 23 Portland Place, London, W1N 3AS tel: 01-637 7181.

Harder to cope with is the situation where a nurse visits but has an unacceptable attitude. The first thing to do is to talk to the supervisor and explain the position as fully and coolly as you can. Then get in touch with your local helpline or AIDS information service to report what has happened. They may be able to make formal representations about what has happened, and they will be able to warn other people of potential problems.

Help through social workers

A social worker can help and advise on a very wide range of problems, including practical, emotional and financial questions. A social worker who is unable to help directly should be able to tell you who can. Most social workers are based in the social services departments of local authorities. To get in contact phone (ask for the duty officer), visit or write. In some areas there are social workers who have special responsibility for people with AIDS and their carers, or may even work with a special home care team – see page 62. In some areas you may find social workers are severely overstretched:

There aren't enough social workers, I got one by ringing the area manager before the weekly allocation meeting and insisted that it was an emergency

Some social workers work from health centres and may be particularly useful when someone frequently uses the health centre or a GP based in it. Social workers based in hospitals may help ease the problems of leaving hospital by making sure that community social workers know what is needed and that there is some continuity of care. They will be particularly useful for people who have frequent stays in hospital followed by periods at home. Social workers will tell you about the other services the local authority offers, and may be able to arrange for them. These include:

Occupational therapists

Occupational therapists (OTs) help with the tasks of everyday living – bathing, dressing, cooking and eating, for example – by teaching people new ways of doing things they have difficulty with, or by advising on or providing special equipment to make these things easier. There are over 3000 devices which are designed to make everyday tasks easier. They include bath seats and rails, raised toilet seats, gadgets which make washing, dressing, cooking or using common household items such as the telephone easier. Occupational therapists will also advise on any structural alterations which may help, particularly if someone has problems of mobility. They are also able to instruct people who are ill in new ways of carrying out everyday activities. Those who work from social service departments visit their clients at home. Others work in hospitals. If your local social service department does not employ an OT, a social worker may help directly or pass you on to the health authority, which will in some areas be able to provide equipment. Or you can ask your doctor to refer you to the consultant at the nearest hospital with an OT department.

. . . got us sticks and a wheelchair and we took him out. It made him feel one hundred per cent better

Home helps

Home helps (sometimes called *home care, domiciliary care* or *community care* aides or assistants) are employed by social service departments. They may help with domestic duties such as housework, shopping and preparing meals. They aim to create a supportive homely atmosphere where clients can achieve maximum independence. They may wash clothes and bedlinen too (but see below if frequent changes of bedclothes are needed). In some areas home helps may be trained to help with simple nursing duties.

If you want a home help get in touch with the social worker. The home help organiser will usually visit to make a preliminary assessment. To avoid any misunderstanding check with the organiser what the home help will and won't do, how often and for how long he/she will be able to visit and whether any charges are involved. In some areas the home help service is free; in others, depending on financial position, there will be a fee. In some areas there aren't enough home helps and it may be difficult to get one. Explain clearly why you particularly need help and try to get your GP to support your request.

Meals on Wheels

Meals on Wheels can deliver hot meals by arrangement with the social service department if cooking is a problem. You may not be able to arrange for these to be supplied every day; some areas have a weekend service for people in particular need – ask your social services department.

Adaptations

If a house or flat is really unsuitable for someone who becomes ill, it may be possible to get financial help towards adapting it. Occupational therapists advise on alterations which may solve immediate problems – see page 54.

Laundry service

In some areas the social services department runs a laundry service, usually for people who are incontinent and need frequent changes of bedlinen. In some cases it may accept other laundry from people who are too ill to do their own washing. In some areas this service will be run by the health authority. In either case ask your GP, district nurse or social services department for details. (There is usually a fee for this service.)

If you need a washing machine (or other equipment which would make life easier) see page 176 for details of the various charities which give money for these purposes. See also details of the Family Fund on page 162.

Services set up for people with AIDS

The main organisations are described in this chapter and in appropriate chapters elsewhere in this book. A list of some local helplines is given on page 295. Local organisations may offer a variety of services such as befriending, counselling, buddying. home care, support groups and various other kinds of practical help. For more information, including the address and telephone number of your local helpline, contact the National AIDS Helpline, Terrence Higgins Trust, Scottish Aids Monitor, or the AIDS helpline in Northern Ireland – see below for details of all these.

The National AIDS Helpline

The National AIDS Helpline keeps up-to-date information about all organisations and individuals who provide any kind of service related to HIV, ARC or AIDS. As new services are being set up all the time, and the situation can change fast in this field, it is *always* worth checking with the Helpline for the latest list of relevant groups. Phone calls are free from anywhere in the UK and you can phone at any time: (0800) 567 123

Advice and literature is also available in the following languages:
Arabic languages: (0800) 282 447 (6pm to 10pm on Wednesdays);
Asian languages: (0800) 282 445 (6pm to 10pm on Wednesdays);
Cantonese: (0800) 282 446 (6pm to 10pm on Tuesdays).

Minicom service (a bit like Telex) for people who are hard of hearing: (0800) 521 361 (10am to 10pm every day).

A leaflets hotline, the Health Literature Line, will send you free leaflets and books (it does *not* keep a record of people who ask for them): PO Box 1577, London NW1 3DW (0800) 555 777

The National AIDS Manual

It may be worth checking if the helpline or advice service you are using subscribes to the National AIDS Manual. It provides information on a comprehensive range of issues, provides answers to questions people often ask, and has a full list of all the organisations which provide information and services relating to any aspect of HIV. The manual is for agencies and health advisors involved in HIV work rather than individuals. (It costs £195 for the first year, or £55 for voluntary organisations, to include two updates.) If the helpline or service *does* subscribe you can be pretty sure that the information it gives you is up-to-date.

NAM Publications Ltd
PO Box 99
London SW2 1EL   01-737 1846

The Terrence Higgins Trust

The Terrence Higgins Trust (THT) is the main organisation in England and Wales for information, advice and support relating to HIV, ARC or AIDS. Their *Helpline* gives advice, information and help to anyone on any aspect of HIV or AIDS. Calls are answered by trained counsellors. The Helpline also has specialists who give advice on *welfare rights* (social security, debt, entitlement to local authority services). They will be able to give you details of your nearest local source of advice. Advice on *legal matters* is given by lawyers on the Legal Line. Also see page 93 for basic information on legal matters.

The THT also have a number of support groups. Contact them for up-to-date information about groups for people with AIDS and those for partners, families and friends. Details of the Family Support Network are given on page 277; see page 278 for information about the Lovers' Support Group, and page 262 for information about a group for people who have lost a partner. Details of the 'buddy' system are given on page 68.

Face-to-face counselling is given by a team of trained counsellors to anyone who needs it. These include people who have been newly diagnosed as HIV-positive, people learning to live with AIDS, carers, friends, the 'worried well' and professional workers in the field. Most counselling is carried out at the THT although counsellors will visit hospitals on occasion. If you need counselling you can usually be seen within a few days of contacting the THT.

Other services include counselling, information and services for drug users, prison liaison, campaigning and information-giving of many kinds. (See page 263 for details of the Interfaith religious group.)

The THT *Library* has the UK's largest collection of books and audio-visual materials on the non-medical aspects of HIV. Anyone is welcome to use the library, provided an appointment is made. Books cannot be borrowed. Contact the librarian for more information.

The THT have a number of leaflets and other publications – contact them for up-to-date details. (See page 182 for details of funds to help people facing hardship.)

52-54 Gray's Inn Road
London WC1X 8LT   01-831 0330
Helpline – 01-242 1010 (3pm to 10pm every day)

For Vistel (phones connected to a screen so information can be given in text form), ring 01-405 2463 (7pm to 10pm every day). This system will soon be replaced by Minicom. Legal Line – 01-405 2381 (7pm to 10pm on Wednesdays).

Scottish AIDS Monitor (SAM)

In Scotland, SAM provides information, counselling and support, including legal advice, information on safe sex and drug use and on any other HIV-related subject. Their main offices are in Edinburgh and Glasgow.

> Edinburgh 031-557 1757 (7.30pm to 10pm, every day)
> Glasgow 041-221 7467 (7pm to 10pm, Tuesdays, Wednesdays, Thursdays)
> Aberdeen (0224) 574000 (7pm to 10pm, Tuesdays, Fridays)

Advice on welfare rights (income support, disability and housing benefits, for example) is given by the welfare rights officer at Glasgow (Mondays and Thursdays), Edinburgh (Tuesdays and Fridays) and at the Counselling Clinic, Ruchill Hospital, Glasgow, on Wednesdays. See page 69 for details of SAM's Buddy Scheme and details of Body Positive groups in Edinburgh and Glasgow.

> SAM
> National Office
> PO Box 48
> Edinburgh EH1 5SA
> 031-557 3885
>
> SAM
> Glasgow Office
> PO Box 111
> Glasgow G2 2UT
> 041-204 1127

The AIDS Helpline (Northern Ireland)

This is the main voluntary AIDS organisation in the province. They helped set up a Body Positive group (see page 59) based in Belfast and organise buddying, working closely with the Eastern Health and Social Services Board Aids steering group. Together they have developed education programmes for health and social workers, and the public. They are setting up support for both people with AIDS and their carers. The Helpline offers advice and counselling, and can arrange referrals to hospital and other contacts throughout the province; they can also arrange confidential face-to-face counselling in their office.

> AIDS Helpline (Northern Ireland)
> PO Box 206
> Belfast BT1 1FJ   (0232) 326117
> (7.30 to 10pm, Mondays, Wednesdays, Fridays; 2pm to 5pm, Saturdays).

Self-help groups

Black HIV and AIDS network

The Black HIV and AIDS Network have groups in London, Leicester and Liverpool and hope to establish others elsewhere. They give general information about HIV and AIDS, offer practical support to black people and counselling face-to-face or by phone.

> Black HIV and AIDS Network
> BM MCC
> London WC1N 3XX   01-485 6756

Blackliners

Blackliners run a Helpline staffed by trained counsellors who give advice to black and Asian people about HIV, AIDS and drug addiction. They can also arrange face-to-face counselling during the day. They hope to set up support groups and buddy schemes in the near future. The Helpline is open from 1pm to 4pm Tuesday to Friday:

> Blackliners
> PO Box 74
> London SW12 9JY   01-673 1695

Body Positive

Body Positive was set up as a self-help group for people who are HIV-positive. They will give advice, support and practical help to anyone on any issue related to HIV. There are other Body Positive groups in London and throughout the country – the main London office has details. Their telephone helpline is answered by people who are HIV-positive themselves. They will give you information and advice directly, or arrange for face-to-face counselling.

They aim to help people use their own strengths to meet the individual challenges they face. Their newsletter – *BP News* – comes out every two weeks, and gives news about HIV-related issues, results of the latest research into HIV, information on staying healthy, details of social events and so on. It has a page of personal advertisements covering details of contacts, accommodation and services.

They also organise information weekends for anyone concerned – people with AIDS themselves, family, friends, representatives of organisations, for example. The weekend includes discussions on living with HIV from the point of view of the person with HIV, carer, partner and family; diet; exercise and ways of remaining in optimum health and other issues related to HIV such as bereavement and grief. Charges to individuals are made to cover food only – around £9.

A support group for people with an HIV infection (and their carers) is held by Body Positive at the London Lesbian and Gay Centre (67-69 Cowcross Street, London EC1) every Sunday. On the third Sunday of every month a talk is given – with discussion – on HIV and AIDS at The Kobler Centre at St Stephen's Hospital, Fulham Road, London SW6.

For anyone living in London who needs personal contact – or just someone to talk to – Body Positive will arrange for someone who is HIV-positive to visit. They have a visiting service for people in hospital and run a daytime drop-in centre – see page 66. Body Positive also have a grants fund – see page 178.

Body Positive
51b Philbeach Gardens
London SW5 9EB
Helpline 01-373 9124 (7pm to 10pm, Monday to Friday).

Frontliners

Frontliners UK Ltd are a registered charity. They are a self-help group organised and run solely by people with AIDS. They provide both emotional and practical support. Advice, counselling and education is given by people who speak from personal experience and explain how AIDS can be controlled and lived with. Practical support is given in a number of ways, including money (see page 179), information, liaison with other helping agencies, and ensuring that people get all available appropriate help. They aim to give special help to the newly diagnosed.

Frontliners have a number of healthcare projects aimed at finding better ways of staying healthy, using either conventional or complementary therapies or both. Their book *Living with AIDS: A Guide to Survival by People with AIDS* costs £9.95 (proceeds go to help people with AIDS and ARC) but is free to those with AIDS or ARC. They also have a newsletter called *Frontiers*.

Frontliners share a headquarters with the THT, and can be contacted from 10am to 4.30pm on weekdays on the THT number (01-831 0330) or, failing that, on a direct line – 01-404 4324 – which has an answerphone outside office hours. The direct line is fitted with a Minicom for people who are hard of hearing.

In London, branches of Frontliners are being set up at St Mary's, Middlesex and Westminster hospitals, in Mildmay Mission Hospital, London Lighthouse and elsewhere. Other branches are being set up in other parts of the country – contact one of the numbers below for the latest information. Frontliners is a national organisation and you will get help no matter where you live.

Frontliners UK Ltd
52-54 Gray's Inn Road
London WC1X 8JU   01-831 0330 (or 01-404 4324 if there is difficulty).

Frontliners Scottish Division
37-39 Montrose Terrace
Edinburgh EH7 5DJ   031-652 0754

Positive Partners

Positive Partners is a self-help group open to anybody who is HIV-positive or who has ARC or AIDS, and to partners and family members. They hold regular meetings, where people can talk freely and easily about whatever is most important to them at the time. Sometimes this may be about HIV, at other times about health, relationships, trying to give up drugs or other subjects. The groups are friendly and informal – there are no leaders. Anyone affected directly or indirectly by HIV is welcome to attend – irrespective of lifestyle, colour, race, religion, sexual orientation or anything else. Positive Partners also have a 24-hour telephone helpline. Groups are being established in various parts of London, Edinburgh, Southampton and Swansea. Positive Partners will be able to tell you about any new groups.

Positive Partners
10 Rathbone Place
London W1   01-249 6068

The Aled Richards Trust

The Aled Richards Trust is a charity set up specifically to help people with HIV or AIDS. Their telephone helpline gives advice to anyone concerned about HIV, and provides face-to-face counselling to anyone affected by the virus – people with AIDS, their carers, partners and families. They also have a buddying service, a support group – Positively Close – for family, friends, partners and carers, and a Holistic Health Group which organises courses on diet, yoga, relaxation and so on. They can arrange referrals to complementary medicine practitioners. Their gay men's, drug-users' and women's groups co-ordinate information and education on HIV-related issues. They also make small grants and loans – see page 177.

> The Aled Richards Trust
> 54 Colston Street
> Bristol BS1 5AZ   (0272) 297963 (Office)
> Helpline: (0272) 273436 (7pm to 9pm, Mondays to Fridays).

Help for women

See page 221 for details of Positively Women.

Home care teams

Some hospitals and local authorities have set up, or are in the process of setting up, special home care teams. These may provide services directly for people with AIDS at home or may co-ordinate existing hospital community and medical services. Check with a helpline for more up-to-date information.

London

Bloomsbury Community Care Team
This consists of a consultant in palliative medicine, two senior nurses, a social worker, administrator and research assistant, and has advisors on occupational therapy and diet. The team helps with pain and symptom control, emotional and spiritual matters and provides education, advice and liaison with health and social workers and voluntary organisations. They give a direct service to people with AIDS at home who either live in Bloomsbury or are patients of the Middlesex or University College Hospitals.

> Community Care Team
> National Temperance Hospital
> Hampstead Road
> London NW1 2LT   01-380 9760

Middlesex Hospital
A team of five health advisors are based in the genito-urinary clinic and sees people as out-patients. They do not make home visits but liaise with community medical and social services. Three specialist psychologists give counselling from the same clinic. An HIV social worker and a drug services social worker are employed in the hospital and also work in the community.

Home Support Team, St Mary's Hospital, Paddington, London
The Home Support Team is composed of six nurses, a GP and a welfare rights

officer. They provide a continuing service for anyone with HIV infection or AIDS who needs care. With consent, they refer people to the relevant community and hospital services and provide direct help where necessary. They also run a local support group for carers. Tel 01-725 1570

Westminster Hospital
The HIV liaison sister, occupational therapist and social worker are responsible for co-ordinating hospital and community care, assessing a patient's needs and making sure that they are being met. The team does not provide services directly.

Westminster Social Services Home Care Team
Ten staff provide a seven-days-a-week service for people in Westminster, giving practical help and a buddy service.

London Lighthouse
London Lighthouse (see also page 71) supply a home support service for people in London, using a team of trained volunteers. They offer non-medical nursing care and support, depending on individual needs. In some cases 12- or 24-hour support may be given on a rota basis; other people may only need a few hours a week. 'Nightlights' is a care group of volunteers who are able to stay overnight. If necessary 24-hour care can be provided. The Home Support Organiser makes an initial visit to make sure the service can provide what is needed, and will also be there when the volunteer first visits. For information contact the Community Services Department – 01-792 1200.

Brighton

The Home Care Support Team is based at the Sussex AIDS Centre and Helpline and run by them in conjunction with the Brighton Health Authority. They work with people who are terminally ill and those who need convalescent care after acute hospital treatment. Their aim is to enable those who wish to live at home to do so. The team consists of four registered nurses, four home care workers, supplemented by volunteers.

Sussex AIDS Centre and Helpline
PO Box 17
Brighton BN2 5NQ   (0273) 608511 (office hours).
Helpline – see page 301.

Edinburgh

Discharge arrangements from hospital are co-ordinated by a social worker, occupational therapist and a community nurse, bringing together statutory agencies and voluntary groups.

Positive Help

In Edinburgh and Lothian Positive Help provides practical help for people who are HIV-positive, or have ARC or AIDS, and their families, friends and carers. They don't offer counselling, but trained volunteers offer practical help such as decorating homes or transporting people to hospital, and are willing to talk.

> Positive Help
> 7 Upper Bow
> Edinburgh EH1 2JN   031-220 3975 (mornings best).

Glasgow

In Strathclyde, people with AIDS living at home use home care services provided by the Social Work Department and the Health Boards.

A counselling clinic team based in the Infectious Diseases Unit at Ruchill Hospital advise, train and support social and health care workers, and co-ordinate services from there and from voluntary organisations. The social workers liaise with services offered throughout the Strathclyde Region. In some cases, to protect confidentiality, services such as home helps will be provided from an adjoining area. Health workers include community nurses, occupational therapists, a drug worker and a senior psychologist. They co-ordinate services within Glasgow, but patients may come to Ruchill from any of the Health Board areas.

Support services are also available from the counselling clinic itself. These include individual, family and group counselling and therapy as well as self-help groups for people with HIV or AIDS and their partners and families.

> The Counselling Clinic
> Ruchill Hospital
> Bilsland Drive
> Glasgow G20 9NB
> 041-946 7120 (hospital no. – 24 hours)
> 041-946 5247 (clinic – 9am to 5pm Monday to Friday).

Newcastle

The Community Support Team is a group of experienced people including a nurse adviser, social work counsellor, clinical psychologist and community worker, who arrange and provide direct care and support to people with HIV infection, their carers, partners and families. Where possible, they enable patients to live outside the hospital. They arrange help with physical care, emotional support, and help with the psychological, practical, financial and other difficulties that can arise from living with HIV. They also offer consultation, training, support and advice on matters relating to HIV and AIDS.

> Community Support Centre
> 52 Clifton Road
> Newcastle-upon-Tyne
> NE4 8DQ   091-273 0197

Oxford

OXAIDS

OXAIDS run a voluntary support service for people who need help with things like shopping, cleaning and transport. They also have a buddying service. If you want help, get in touch with the Development Worker at: OXAIDS Helpline (0865) 728817 (11am to 7pm on weekdays).

National

ACET (Aids Care Education and Training)

ACET is a charity which uses volunteers (supported and trained by nurses) to help people with AIDS stay at home if they wish. At present the majority of volunteers are in London and Scotland, but they aim to have a volunteer within an hour's drive of anyone in the UK. A nurse makes an assessment and plans the level of support required. Volunteers provide practical help such as shopping, cleaning and transport to and from hospital. There is also a night-sitting service. ACET nurses can advise and liaise with GPs, community and medical services. Volunteers can call on a team of doctors, nurses and social workers at any time. These services are free, and any information given to ACET is confidential. Phone between 9am and 5pm Monday to Friday. ACET also gives grants to people with special needs – see page 176.

PO Box 1323	PO Box 108
London W5 5TF	Edinburgh EH8 9NY
01-840 7879	031-668 4225
PO Box 147	PO Box 153
Portsmouth PO2 9DA	Dundee DD1 9RH
(0705) 693422	(0382) 202463

Day centres

Day centres are places where people with HIV can go during the day. They make it possible to continue living at home even when a considerable amount of care is needed, and enable carers to continue working. The day centres which have so far been set up for people with AIDS offer different kinds of service but all are non-institutional, welcoming and pleasant.

The Body Positive Centre

The Body Positive Centre is intended to be a safe and welcoming place for anyone affected by HIV or AIDS. Both professional and informal counselling are available, as well as information and advice on welfare rights and housing. The Centre provides facilities (for example, there is a library of information on HIV and AIDS), opportunities for daytime and evening activities (such as in art and creative writing). They are a base for several organised groups. A basic midday meal can be had at reasonable cost. (See also page 59.)

> Body Positive Centre
> 51b Philbeach Gardens
> London SW5 9EB   01-835 1045

The Kobler Centre

The Centre is attached to St Stephen's Hospital in Fulham, London. It has an out-patients' clinic and day-care facilities for such things as monitoring of drugs, blood transfusions and minor surgery which doesn't require overnight admission. Doctors can be seen without making an appointment, and routine check-ups can be made at the centre without going into the hospital itself. Also available are counselling, a social worker, health advisor, dietitian, physiotherapist and occupational therapist. People with AIDS are welcome to bring friends.

> The Kobler Centre
> St Stephen's Clinic
> St Stephen's Hospital site
> Corner of Netherton Grove and Fulham Road
> London SW10 9HT   01-376 4555

Landmark

This is a walk-in centre for South London. It offers free weekly advice to anyone affected by HIV with sessions on money, the law, housing, nursing for carers and diet. Facilities include food, cooking and laundry, a library, massage and acupuncture sessions. Landmark can also arrange transport where needed.

> 47a Tulse Hill
> London SW2 2TN   01-678 6686

The London Lighthouse

The Lighthouse provides a meeting place for people with AIDS, their partners, friends and families. There are lounges, a cafe, and seating in a garden. A shop stocking books, videos and tapes is planned. Counselling is available on a drop-in basis (from 9.30am to 4.30pm each day) as well as by appointment, and there are weekly support groups (for gay men, women, ex-drug users, people who have been newly diagnosed, partners, parents and relatives, for example) and art and music classes. The Lighthouse also runs a series of health workshops and information courses: these include health programmes aimed at enabling people to make informed decisions about diet, exercise and relaxation as well as providing information about orthodox and complementary medicine. There is usually a fee although a number of assisted places for people with HIV are available. The London Lighthouse is open seven days a week – see page 71 for more information.

> 111/117 Lancaster Road
> London W11 1QT   01-792 1200

The Sussex AIDS Centre and Helpline

The Centre in Brighton has a sitting room, kitchen and a quiet area. Body Positive (see page 59) hold group meetings there, and counselling is available (it's best to phone first and make an appointment).

> Sussex AIDS Centre and Helpline
> PO Box 17
> Brighton
> BN2 5NQ
> (0273) 608511 (Office)
> (0273) 571660 (Helpline 8pm to 10pm).

Drop in centres

Those running at the time of writing are listed below; for up-to-date information contact your local AIDS Helpline.

> London: Ealing Hounslow and Ealing AIDS Response Service 01-571 9191
> Hastings: Hastings and Rother AIDS Support Society (0424) 429901
> Hull: Hull Aids Action (0482) 27060
> St Albans and Hemel Hempstead: The Crescent – HIV/AIDS Information and Counselling Centre 0727 44230 (St Albans) 0442 42942 (Hemel Hempstead).

Buddy schemes

Buddy schemes were pioneered in the USA and have now become one of the principal ways of providing support for people with ARC or AIDS. Below we describe the scheme organised by the Terrence Higgins Trust, which is the most developed in the country. The SAM scheme in Scotland is similar.

A buddy is a person who is there to provide whatever support the person with AIDS needs. His or her role will vary according to the wishes and needs of each individual. This may consist of practical things – doing some shopping or cleaning, liaising with other people – or just being there. But the main aim of a buddy is to enable people with AIDS to make their own decisions and achieve the highest possible quality of life. Buddies do not take the place of or do the work of anyone else, and should not be seen as a threat to any existing relationship. Partners have sometimes needlessly become suspicious of buddies who become close to the person with AIDS. In fact buddies often have the important role of being an independent listener, outside the relationship between the person with AIDS and their partner.

x and y communicated better when the buddy was there, and acted as a catalyst in getting them to discuss things.

. . . they're very quarrelsome together – I'm in the middle, a buffer.

One buddy felt that a total stranger can be easier for a person with AIDS to talk to, particularly as 'you need to get rid of secrets'; talk about bad relationships, abuse suffered as a child and things it might be difficult to discuss with someone known well.

Buddies are not chosen because they have any one particular skill but do go through a careful process of selection and training. All buddies are committed and will give support for as long as is needed; they will keep in regular contact (at least once a week) and not let anyone down by suddenly disappearing. Although buddies are often active people with a full-time job and a full social life they are able to give the person with AIDS more time and personal attention than many professionals. Conversely, buddies are able to recognise times when they are not needed and do not feel threatened or unhappy about this in the way a long-standing friend might. Sometimes buddies can give support to partners and other carers after someone has died, if needed; this continuity can be very important.

The buddy service is free and absolutely confidential. There are about 170 THT buddies in London, and this number is increasing. About a third of them are women. They are supported by follow-up training sessions, which take place four times a year, and by their own groups which meet every month. Additionally, for mainly practical help, they can call on *helper cells* – people who help with one-off tasks.

If the person you are caring for wants a buddy the THT should be contacted as early as possible. The area co-ordinator will visit to find out more. After this a buddy will be allocated. A priority system exists to make sure urgent needs are met quickly. But note that THT buddies are there to help people with ARC or AIDS and do not usually give support to other people with HIV. In Scotland SAM can provide buddies for people who are HIV-positive as well.

Some buddy schemes outside London, are run on the same lines, particularly as many organisers have attended THT courses. If your local scheme is different it may be worth finding out about what they do, what training has been given and so on. Well-established schemes exist in Edinburgh and Glasgow (with about 80 buddies in each) and there may be one in Dundee soon – information from the counselling and training officer at Scottish AIDS Monitor in Edinburgh or Glasgow (addresses on page 58).

Hospices

Hospices are a comparatively recent development. They were originally set up to look after people in the last stages of an incurable disease, who can no longer be helped by medical treatment. Their underlying philosophy is that a dying patient is a living patient. Their aim is to provide dignity, security, calm and fulfilment in the last stages of life. They provide help with controlling pain and distressing symptoms, and try to meet the emotional and other needs of patients and their families. To do this they employ specially trained staff; it is not unusual to find one member of staff for every hospice patient. Hospices have doctors, nurses, social workers and other staff on hand, and can arrange to call on any skills needed to make a patient as comfortable as possible. Most hospice patients have some form of cancer, and some have motor neurone disease.

At the end of 1989 there were over 130 hospice in-patient units in the UK, and Ireland which, between them, looked after more than 25,000 people each year. Typically, patients are admitted towards the very end of their lives, when they can no longer be looked after at home.

Hospices will continue to give help and support to relatives and friends after a bereavement, for as long as is necessary. Each hospice is autonomous; they are all run in slightly different ways and have different criteria for admission. Some will take people with AIDS, some will do so only if the person has an illness (such as cancer) which the hospice is used to dealing with. Some hospices receive the majority of their funding from cancer charities and so can accept only a certain number of people who do not have cancer. A minority of hospices do not accept people with AIDS at all, but this is expected to become increasingly rare. Hospices are unlikely to accept people who are drug users.

Although the majority of people admitted to hospices are elderly, all hospices have admitted young people from time to time, and can provide the kind of support and help they need. Elderly people in hospices are often extremely grateful for the help they are given, while younger people who are dying sometimes show a considerable amount of anger and other strong feelings. This may also be true of people with AIDS and it is reasonably safe to expect the hospice to be able to cope sympathetically with this. Often people with AIDS will be nursed in private rooms in hospices. You can visit patients in hospices as often and for as long as you like, at any time of the day or evening. Hospices do all they can to avoid an 'institutional' feel.

Although a small number are run by the NHS, others are run by voluntary organisations or are charities in their own right. Hospices usually do not charge, but some independent hospices who receive no money from the NHS may be dependent on voluntary contributions. Hospices never refuse to admit someone just because they cannot pay.

People can be referred to a hospice by doctors, nurses or any other health or social workers, or you can get in touch directly. Generally, hospices will take people who live in the Health District in which they are situated, or up to the catchment area of a neighbouring hospice. Hospices tend to be full most of the time, and reckon just to keep pace with the demand. It may be particularly hard to find space in some areas, such as London, and it is not generally possible to arrange admission in hospices outside the home area unless there are strong family links with that area. It is wise to go and see the hospice beforehand, and talk to as many of the key staff as you can.

Your GP, social worker, local library or CAB should be able to tell you where your nearest hospice is. Otherwise you can get a list from:

> The Hospice Information Service
> St Christopher's Hospice
> 51/59 Lawrie Park Road
> Sydenham
> London SE26 6DZ   01-778 9252

General information about the hospice movement can be obtained from:

> Help the Hospices
> BMA House
> Tavistock Square
> London WC1H 9JP   01-388 7807/0649

At the time of writing only two hospices have been set up specifically to help people with AIDS. Both of them are in London, although they will accept people from anywhere in the country.

London Lighthouse

London Lighthouse was built to provide a welcoming and pleasant place for anyone concerned about HIV. It has a cafe, drop-in centre and many other services. See page 67 for details of these.

The residential unit is designed to be comfortable and uninstitutional. It is both for people who will remain for the duration of their illness as well as for those who need or want to stay only for a short time. Appropriate care can be given to those who need to convalesce for a limited time, those who are learning to keep symptoms under control and those who need care in the last stages of an illness. It will particularly help people who:

- are convalescing from a serious illness, and are not yet able to go home
- need some care, but whose usual carers need a break
- do not need the kind of medical treatment that hospitals provide, but do need nursing and simple medical care
- have practical difficulties which mean they can no longer be nursed at home.

London Lighthouse is open to anyone in the country – you don't have to be or have been living in London to qualify. Applications can be made by a person with AIDS direct, or, with his or her permission, by a carer, GP, hospital staff or community worker. Each application will be considered and it is intended that places will be given solely on the basis of need, limited by the number of beds available. For more information get in touch with the Residential Unit. The Lighthouse also has a support service for people with AIDS or ARC which aims to enable them to live independently at home – see page 63.

London Lighthouse
111–117 Lancaster Road
London W11 1QT   01-792 1200

Mildmay Mission Hospital

The Mildmay Mission Hospital is an independent Christian charitable hospital which, among other things, provides facilities for young disabled people. In February 1988 it opened the first hospice unit specifically for people with AIDS. Mildmay is staffed mostly by Christians who accept and care for patients regardless of race, creed, culture or lifestyle.

Mildmay will take people for short periods of up to four weeks to give regular carers a break, or for periods of convalescence or rehabilitation; they also accept those who need terminal care. The care is provided by a team including medical, nursing, counselling, social work, occupational and physiotherapy staff. There is a resident chaplain for those who seek spiritual support. Like all hospices, Mildmay does not have the facilities to offer acute medical care. They give treatment aimed at controlling and minimising symptoms and enhancing the quality of life. For patients who are dying they aim to make this as peaceful, comfortable and dignified as possible. Bereavement counselling and support is also offered to carers throughout and beyond this period.

There are seventeen single rooms, each furnished to be as like home as possible; residents are encouraged to bring their own bits and pieces. Each has a bedchair, so that partners and friends are able to stay. Other facilities include kitchen, dining area, roof garden, communal and family room. A Day Centre and a home care team started operation in November 1989. A new unit will provide care for mothers with HIV and their babies. Mildmay accept people from all over the country. Each is considered according to need and urgency. Referral is through a GP or consultant.

Mildmay Mission Hospital
Hackney Road
London E2 7NA   01-739 2331

The Waverley Care Trust plan facilities for residential nursing, midterm respite and hospice care in Edinburgh (from mid 1990) and Glasgow (1991). Phone 031-220 4697 for details. See page 235 for future facilities for drug users.

Other voluntary organisations

Organisations set up for people with cancer
BACUP

BACUP is a free national cancer information service which helps cancer patients and their families live with cancer by providing the latest information, practical advice and emotional support. A team of specially trained and experienced cancer nurses, supported by a panel of medical specialists, answer enquiries by telephone or letter about any aspect of cancer. They currently receive over 500 enquiries a week.

A wide range of clearly written and illustrated booklets, covering specific types of cancer, their treatments and other related topics, are sent free to those who use the service. A newsletter is produced three times a year.

While they focus entirely on cancer and may not have general information relevant to HIV, BACUP can give useful information about chemotherapy and radiotherapy, including side effects and how to deal with them. From their resource directory of over 2,000 references, they can provide information about local support groups, but you should get in touch with an individual group to find out if they could give appropriate help.

BACUP
121/123 Charterhouse Street
London EC1M 6AA
Cancer Information Service 01-608 1661 (10am to 7pm, Mondays to Thursdays; 10am to 5.30pm, Fridays)
Freephone for people outside London (0800) 181199

Cancer Link

Cancer Link are a charity which provides information and services for people with cancer, their family and friends. Their nurses can give information by phone or letter on treatment, as well as practical or emotional help including visiting, and will give details of any local cancer support and self-help groups. Some groups specialise in certain forms of cancer or in particular treatments or therapies including complementary medicine. Cancer Link publish a directory of these groups, describing the activities of each; it costs £2 including p+p from:

Cancer Link
17 Britannia Street   9 Castle Terrace
London WC1X 9JN   01-833 2451   Edinburgh EH1 2DP   031-228 5557

General

In most areas local groups exist to provide all kinds of help – shopping, gardening, decorating and any other task which has become difficult. These have not been set up specifically to help with HIV. We cannot tell you precisely what will be available locally, nor whether individual local branches are broadly sympathetic to the situation of those with HIV-related illnesses.

To find out what is available get in touch with your local Council for Voluntary Service (sometimes called Council of Social Service or Guild of Social Welfare), or the Rural Community Council in rural areas. Addresses can be found in your phone book, library, CAB or from the National Council for Voluntary Organisations (NCVO) – send a stamped addressed envelope to:

NCVO Information and Intelligence Unit
26 Bedford Square
London WC1B 3HU   01-636 4066

The British Red Cross

While the British Red Cross do not have a specific service for people with AIDS and their carers, they organise various local services which may be useful.

Home nursing
British Red Cross volunteers help with some basic nursing services, such as washing and bathing and dealing with incontinence, as well as help with visiting and shopping. An assessment visit is made first. British Red Cross volunteers organise their work in conjunction with services provided by other volunteers and the health and social services. However, when someone does not want any other services to be involved, the Red Cross nurse will respect these wishes. Their availability varies from area to area.

Cosmetic camouflage programme
Lesions caused by Kaposi's sarcoma and other skin rashes cause huge distress if they appear in easily visible places. Red Cross consultants teach people how to cover these up with special make-up, and will provide the materials needed. The Red Cross say that this is usually effective, even for those with a considerable number of lesions, with tremendous psychological benefit. Tuition has to be arranged through a doctor and usually takes place in hospital, although a service in your own home may be available soon.

Transport and escorts
The Red Cross provide a transport service (but not in Scotland) for trips to and from hospital or for any other purpose, including longer journeys between cities (and even, to other countries). Transport is mostly by ambulance which, if necessary can be fitted out to cope with the medical needs of the passenger. The Red Cross have a scale of charges, based on distance, for this service. If you are using public or private transport the Red Cross can provide a trained volunteer as an escort. There is no charge for this, although you have to pay the escort's fares. Some notice is needed for this service. The *medical loan service* can lend equipment such as walking frames and commodes. They can also supply equipment to help deal with incontinence. There may be a small nominal charge for these; the NHS pays most of the cost. Availability varies: check with your local branch.

The British Red Cross Society
9 Grosvenor Crescent
London SW1X 7EJ   01-235 5454

The WRVS

The Women's Royal Voluntary Service work both independently and with health and local authority services. Work is carried out by volunteers; most, but not all, are women.

Services vary from area to area but may include shopping, collecting prescriptions, supplying clothing and bedding, and providing escorts. They may also have a sitting service for carers who need a few hours' break and be able to help with transport, using their volunteers' own cars. The WRVS give help only when asked. The address of your local group is in the phone book, or from

WRVS
234–244 Stockwell Road
London SW9 9SP   01-733 3388

Rotary Clubs

Rotary Clubs are made up of business and professional people who offer practical services to the community. Each Club is independent although the central office provides regular information and guidance. Rotarians may be able and willing to give practical help. They are not usually listed in the phone book so ask at your local library or CAB or get in touch with:

Rotary International in Great Britain and Ireland
Kinwarton Road
Alcester
Warwickshire B49 6BP   (0789) 765411 or 01-878 0931

Round Tables

There are over 1,250 Round Tables in the UK, each of which is autonomous. Among other activities they carry out various services for the community in which they are situated. This includes fund-raising for specific projects and for 'round table charities'. It is unlikely that a round table would be able to provide financial assistance but, depending on the policy and priorities of the local group members, may be able to give practical help. To find your nearest Round Table contact:

National Association of Round Tables
Marchesi House
Apex Corner
Birmingham
B2 4QB   021-631 2010

Lions Clubs

There are over 800 Lions Clubs in the UK. Each is independent but all provide practical (such as by providing equipment or transport) or, sometimes, financial help. Each club raises and gives money in its own area. They are listed under Lions in the phone book; otherwise ask at your library, CAB or contact:

Lions Club International Secretariat
5 Vine Terrace
The Square
High Street
Harborne
Birmingham B17 9PU   021-428 1909

Taking things further

People with HIV, friends, family and carers may want to contribute to the fight against AIDS. Many things need to be done.

Campaigning
For better health, social services and information, against discrimination.

Complaining
Against discrimination, misrepresentation in the press or on television.

Contributing time or expertise
Local and national organisations may need help with clerical tasks, secretarial work, fund raising or whatever skills and experience you have. There may be opportunities to be trained to be a 'buddy' (see page 68 for more about 'buddying') or as a counsellor. (For example, the Terrence Higgins Trust run courses in HIV and AIDS counselling. They are held in London and other parts of England. Courses take place over four weekends, spread over four months. A certificate is awarded on completion. THT would also like people with counselling experience to join their volunteer counselling team. For more information

contact the counselling office at THT.) Other national and local organisations may have, or want to develop, all kinds of other services which you could contribute to. Contact the organisation concerned.

Setting up a local organisation
Some areas do not have an AIDS helpline. Many of the self-help organisations described in this book have an expanding network of local groups; you may be able to help start one or contribute to one in your area. Contact the organisation concerned for information. The THT and SAM (see pages 57–8) may also be able to advise.

The National Aids Trust

The National AIDS Trust is a charity which co-ordinates the work of voluntary groups and encourages appropriate new initiatives. If you are thinking of starting a new group they will be able to tell you about any existing groups and any new developments in the pipeline. They may also be able to give practical and financial help – apply to the Grants Administrator.

> The National AIDS Trust
> 14th floor Euston Tower
> 286 Euston Road
> London NW1 3DN   01-388 1188 (x3200)

Network of Voluntary Organisations in AIDS/HIV

NOVOAH is a membership organisation in contact with over 140 voluntary organisations including helplines and self-help groups. They may be able to help with planning and advice.

> NOVOAH
> PO Box 5000
> Glasgow G12 9BL

AIDS Coalition to Unleash Power (ACT-UP)

ACT-UP is an organisation set up to campaign by direct action for the rights of people with HIV, for an end to discrimination against people who have HIV or AIDS and for more government action:

> ACT-UP
> BM Box 2995
> London WC1N 3XX   01-431 4372

Complaining

The basic rules are:

- Complain only when it is necessary – but if it is, make sure that you do. If you don't, things won't change.
- Go to the person you are complaining about first, and give them a chance to sort it out. Some complaints are the result of genuine misunderstandings. Informal complaints may lead to things getting put right without any further bother.
- Make sure you complain to the right person.
- Keep cool.
- Know your facts.
- Complain as soon as it is reasonable to do so.
- A personal visit may be most successful, but follow this up in writing where possible.
- Keep records of everything.
- Don't lose heart.
- Get help where you can. Local AIDS helplines and support groups may be able to help. Also enlist the aid of your Citizens Advice Bureau and other local agencies as appropriate – your library will have details.

Complaints about NHS GPs

The General Medical Council supervises the medical profession, and doctors have to belong to it. Complaints about serious professional misconduct (such as disclosing confidential information inappropriately) should ultimately be made to the GMC. Complaints about poor service or more minor matters should be made to the Medical Services Committee of the Family Practitioner Committee, which is responsible for NHS contracts with GPs.

Registrar
General Medical Council
44 Hallam Street
London W1N 6AE   01-580 7642

Complaints about doctors who treat you privately

Arrangements with private doctors are regarded as contracts. Any complaints about serious professional misconduct should go to the General Medical Council.

Complaints about NHS hospitals and their staff

Complaints about general services should be made to the Hospital Administrator. In serious cases, where professional misconduct is involved, an investigatory tribunal may be set up.

Complaints about clinical judgement (where someone has been wrongly diagnosed, or the practitioner has been negligent in giving treatment, for example) must follow a formal procedure. The first step is to get an appointment with the consultant and ask for an explanation. If this doesn't help write to the Regional Medical Officer at your Health Authority. After discussion the RMO will decide whether the case should be taken any further.

If you are still not satisfied you can contact the Health Service Commissioner (the Ombudsman) for the area in which you live. The Ombudsman cannot investigate complaints which have already been taken to tribunal or court, complaints about clinical judgement or about GPs who are employed under contract by the FPC.

> Health Service Commissioner (Ombudsman) for England
> Church House
> Great Smith Street
> London W1P 3BW   01-276 2035
>
> Northern Ireland Commissioner for Complaints
> 4th floor, Progressive House
> 33 Wellington Place
> Belfast BT1 6HN   (0232) 233821
>
> Health Service Commissioner (Ombudsman) for Scotland
> 2nd floor, 11 Melville Crescent
> Edinburgh EH3 7LU   031-225 7465
>
> Health Service Commissioner (Ombudsman) for Wales
> 4th floor, Pearl Assurance House
> Greyfriars Road
> Cardiff CF1 3AG   (0222) 394621

Community Health Council

The Community Health Council will give you advice and may be able to give practical assistance with any complaints about doctors or the health service. The Citizens Advice Bureau may also be able to help.

Patients Association

The Patients Association is an independent organisation which gives advice and represents patients' interests:

> 18 Victoria Park Square
> Bethnal Green
> London E2 9PF   01-981 5676

Complaints about dentists

Complaints about quality of treatment should go to the Family Practitioners Committee. If the complaint involves professional misconduct you should complain to the General Dental Council.

> General Dental Council
> 37 Wimpole Street
> London W1M 8DQ   01-486 2171

Complaints about welfare benefits

You can appeal against decisions concerning the amount of welfare benefit being paid – see page 172. If you want to complain about the general service (for example about delays in being paid, rudeness or insensitivity on the part of staff) write to the manager. Mark the envelope 'personal' and head the letter 'Letter of Complaint'. If you are not satisfied with the reply you receive, write to the Regional Controller. After this you could contact your MP and the Minister concerned. If your complaint is about maladministration, and you have been unsuccessful in trying to get it resolved by all other means, you can complain as a last resort to the Parliamentary Ombudsman. The matter has to be referred through an MP. You can't involve the Ombudsman if you have already appealed in a Court or tribunal, or could have done so.

4

Counselling

What is counselling?

Counselling aims to help someone identify the main difficulties they face and work out a way of understanding, coping or overcoming them. It may be important to people with HIV, their families, friends and carers, separately or together. This section gives an outline of different kinds of counselling and tells you where to go for more information.

Counsellors are trained to listen and help you come to terms with a problem more clearly. You will have to bring to the counselling session a willingness to spend time with the counsellor and a resolve to be as honest as you can. Counsellors are not threatening in any way, and are easy to talk to – they will not make judgements or blame you for any decisions or actions you have taken or want to take. However, you may find some sessions are very intense if such emotions as pent up anger, frustration, guilt and grief are expressed and discussed. Taking the opportunity to do so in a safe place is a step towards controlling these emotions and reducing the pain they cause.

Counsellors do not make decisions for you or impose their own ideas on you, but help you consider the implications of different courses of action, and then help you carry out the one you choose if you want. If you are having particular difficulties a counsellor may tell you how to overcome the problem so that you can follow a course of action you have both agreed. Counsellors use some psychological techniques and may encourage you to look at aspects of your life and relationships in new ways, or in ways you have not been able to face before.

Your first meeting with a counsellor is likely to be spent in sorting out practical details (such as where and how often to meet, fees and the length of each session). It is also an opportunity to discuss what is likely to be right for you. It may be, after discussion, that you agree that a different course of action would be more helpful, or that you need a counsellor who specialises in a different field. You should feel free to ask any questions you like, so that you can make up your mind about whether you want to work with the counsellor or not. There is no obligation on either side. Any counsellor would expect the first session to be exploratory and should not be offended if you decide not to go ahead. All counselling should be strictly confidential, but you may want to confirm this.

If you do decide to continue, you need to give it a fair trial. Counselling may make you feel worse before you begin to see any benefit. This may be because you are talking about things which are difficult to face up to or because you are gradually coming to terms with the reality of the situation. Sometimes the process of getting to know yourself better can be painful. It will be difficult for you to know if you are making progress, but if you feel you are communicating with a counsellor who understands your situation, the sessions are likely to be productive in the end.

How to find a counsellor

Finding and choosing a counsellor can be tricky. Success can sometimes depend more on personal chemistry than on the counsellor having particular qualifications or depth of experience. However, you should first of all consider finding a counsellor with relevant experience.

Counsellors who specialise in HIV

The following organisations have counsellors experienced in issues related to HIV illness:

Body Positive (page 59)
Positively Women (page 221)
Scottish AIDS Monitor (page 58)
Terrence Higgins Trust (page 57)

Local support groups, local AIDS helplines and lesbian and gay switchboards may also have counsellors experienced in issues related to HIV illnesses. The National AIDS helpline (see page 56) will also give advice over the telephone. In London, both London Lighthouse (page 71) and Mildmay Mission (page 72) have a counselling service. All can give advice on such things as safer sex and other useful information. (See chapter 14 for information on counselling related to drugs and chapter 17 for help during bereavement.) If you find an AIDS counsellor independently (from an advertisement, say) it is worth asking for details of his or her qualifications or experience before you commit yourself.

PACE – Project for Advice Counselling and Education

PACE are based at the London Lesbian and Gay Centre in Farringdon. They counsel lesbians and gay men on any subject including AIDS and HIV, free of charge. This is arranged over several sessions, but there may be a waiting list. Single sessions, likewise on any subject and also free, can be arranged at shorter notice. PACE also give training and advice for groups and organisations. If you are interested in this consider asking your local authority or voluntary organisation to arrange for a course for a group of carers. A reduced rate is charged for voluntary organisations.

PACE
London Lesbian and Gay Centre
67-69 Cowcross Street
London EC1M 6BP   01-251 2689

Clinic 8

AIDS counselling of all kinds is given at Clinic 8 at the Royal Free Hospital in London and by telephone. Sessions are under the direction of a psychologist and family therapist (see page 90 for more information about family therapy). They are experienced in helping people with AIDS, families, partners and carers who have particular worries following diagnosis, those facing bereavement and anyone (including drug-users and children) with HIV-related concerns.

Help can be given by appointment or over the phone, either through the NHS or arranged privately. (If you want to have a long session on the phone you may have to make an appointment to ring at a certain time.) You do not have to live in London to qualify for help, and you do not need to be referred by a doctor.

> Clinic 8, AIDS Counselling Unit
> Royal Free Hospital
> Pond Street
> London NW3 2QG   01-431 0970 (9am to 5pm, Monday to Friday)

St Mary's Hospital

AIDS counselling for people with AIDS and carers is given by clinical psychologists. You can be seen alone or with your partner, or attend one of the information-sharing groups for carers. All sessions are free unless you particularly wish to be seen privately.

> Psychology Department
> Paterson Wing, St Mary's Hospital
> Praed Street
> London W2 1NY   01-725 6542/35

Other sources of counselling

If you are unable to find a counsellor experienced in HIV issues the preliminary interview you have may be particularly important. Counselling is often given informally by GPs, ministers of religion, social workers and other people in the caring professions in the course of their work. Your GP may refer you to a counsellor. Also see page 51 for details of community psychiatric nurses. Outside the NHS, various organisations and individuals offer counselling services. Individual counsellors may have one or more of a number of qualifications as there are many courses and diplomas.

British Association for Counselling

BAC publish the *Counselling and Psychotherapy Resources Directory* each June. It lists individuals who have counselling qualifications and organisations who can supply counsellors, and includes counsellors who aren't members of BAC as well as those who are. It will tell you:

- what qualifications each counsellor has, what kind of counselling they specialise in, whom they counsel (some specialise in particular groups such as married couples, or people who have had a bereavement, for example), and what fees they charge. Fees vary between about £12 and £20 a session, although some are negotiable if you are unable to pay. Some organisations merely ask for a donation, the size of which is up to you.

- which counsellors have experience of counselling related to AIDS, if any. If no counsellor in your area has direct experience, you could look for one who specialises in a similar field.
- which counsellors are BAC-accredited, have passed stringent training requirements and have had substantial practical experience.
- those who work under supervision and have regular contact with an experienced supervisor who can advise them.

The full Directory costs £13.80 (inc p+p) for those who are not members of BAC. However, you can get a free up-to-date copy of the organisations and individual counsellors listed *for your area* by phoning or writing with an SAE to

British Association for Counselling
37a Sheep Street
Rugby
Warwickshire CV21 3BX   (0788) 78328

Scottish Association for Counselling

SAC publish the *Directory of Counselling Services in Scotland* which gives detailed information on over 500 counselling services.

Scottish Association for Counselling
Queen Margaret College
Clerwood Terrace
Edinburgh EH12 8TS   031–339 8111 (x253)
Tuesdays (9.30am to 3.30pm) and Thursdays (9.30am to 12.30pm).

Northern Ireland Association for Counselling

The Northern Ireland Association for Counselling can offer advice on counselling and counsellors within the province, and can supply a list of counsellors and organisations. For AIDS counselling, they advise people to contact the AIDS Helpline Northern Ireland – see page 58.

Northern Ireland Association for Counselling
Bryson House
28 Bedford Street
Belfast BT2 7FE   (0232) 325835 (9am to 1pm, Monday to Friday)

Westminster Pastoral Foundation

The Westminster Pastoral Foundation provide counselling for people who face emotional problems, including those who have a serious or life-threatening illness, who are facing bereavement or who are unhappy, lonely, anxious or depressed for any reason. All counselling is given by trained staff at the Foundation's headquarters in Kensington, London, in affiliated local centres throughout the UK, and to people in their own homes. Group counselling is also given to people who share similar concerns or situations. Counselling for young people (18-24) is organised from the associated Chelsea Pastoral Foundation.

Financial contributions are worked out on a sliding scale and depend on what you are able to afford – nobody is excluded because of a low income. The assessment interview (during which you decide what kind of counselling would be best, how often you should visit and so on) costs up to £30. Individual sessions cost between £5 and £12, and family sessions cost from £15 to £70 a 'family'. Most people have one counselling session a week but you can have them more or less often than this.

Westminster Pastoral Foundation	Chelsea Pastoral Foundation
23 Kensington Square	155a Kings Road
London W8 5HN 01-937 6956	London SW3 5TX 01-351 0839

Psychotherapy

Psychotherapy is similar to counselling, and may use some of the same techniques. It tends to be more intensive and prolonged because it aims to uncover deep-seated psychological reasons for a person's behaviour or personality. Hospital psychotherapists are mostly concerned with psychological disorders and so are not usually an appropriate source of help. Those who practise privately are more likely to accept clients whose needs are not so severe.

British Association of Psychotherapists

The British Association of Psychotherapists offer an initial consultation (£25) to help you decide whether or not psychotherapy is the best form of help for you. If treatment is recommended, a referral to another qualified psychotherapist is arranged. If not, the psychotherapist will usually be able to direct you towards someone else who can help.

> The British Association of Psychotherapists
> 121 Hendon Lane
> London N3 3PR   01-346 1747

Clinical psychologists

Clinical psychologists are graduates in psychology who have taken a two-or three-year course in the application of psychology to health problems. This course includes questions of bereavement, loss, facing up to serious illness and so on.

Clinical psychologists are often able to counsel and advise both people with AIDS and those who care for them. Some may already have experience of HIV and AIDS while others will be familiar with illnesses which may have similar social, medical, financial and emotional consequences. Depending on the area, they are based in hospitals, community mental health departments or there may be a clinical psychology unit in your area. You can get in touch through your GP or the British Psychological Society.

British Psychological Society (BPS)

> St Andrews House
> 48 Princess Road East
> Leicester LE1 7DR   (0533) 549568

The BPS publishes a *Register of Chartered Psychologists* which you should be able to find in the reference section of your local public library.

If you are making direct contact with a clinical psychologist, get in touch with the district psychologist who is responsible for allocating work. Clinical psychologists often have long waiting lists, so you may have to make a case for priority if you need help quickly. It is also worth sounding out the district psychologist to see if anyone has any special expertise which might be particularly helpful – and to get some idea of how sympathetic they are likely to be to your situation.

Family therapy

Institute of Family Therapy

The Institute of Family Therapy (IFT) in London exists to help all members of a 'family' (family means any close relationship – single parent and child, gay or lesbian couple, as well as the traditional nuclear family). Therapy is offered to the whole family together unless it seems helpful or appropriate to see some members separately. Family therapists aim to guide families through periods of crisis or uncertainty. They are experienced in the problems of bereavement and family break-up. The IFT offers therapy sessions at their London premises. Family therapists are to be found in some parts of the country too, but coverage is patchy. The IFT will tell you if there is an IFT-trained or family therapist near you.

> Institute of Family Therapy
> 43 New Cavendish Street
> London W1M 7RG   01-935 1654

Other sources of help

Brook Advisory Centres will advise young people about sexuality and relation-ships. Counselling about relationships is given by Relate and by the Scottish

Marriage Guidance Council (don't be put off by the name – they will also counsel anyone about any relationship). The address should be in your local phone book. Otherwise try:

> Relate (National Marriage Guidance)
> Herbert Gray College
> Little Church Street
> Rugby
> Warwickshire CV21 3AP   (0788) 73241

> Scottish Marriage Guidance Council
> 26 Frederick Street
> Edinburgh EH2 2JR   031-225 5006

See page 221 for details of counselling and advice for children.

Parentline – OPUS is an organisation of Parentline Groups of volunteers who run a telephone helpline for troubled parents; some groups also offer befriending. There are 27 groups in England and Ireland.

> Parentline – OPUS
> 106 Godstone Road
> Whyteleafe
> Surrey CR3 OEB   01-645 0469

National Association of Young People's Counselling and Advisory Services (NAYPCAS)

NAYPCAS is an independent association of local agencies providing counselling, advice and information for young people. Requests from individuals are referred to the appropriate local agency. Counselling and advisory services are provided largely by trained volunteers in centres around the UK. Counselling is usually provided in the agency by appointment or on a call-in basis.

> National Association of Young People's Counselling and Advisory Services (NAYPCAS)
> 17/23 Albion Street
> Leicester LE1 6GD   (0533) 558763

5

Legal matters

HIV and AIDS have posed many legal questions. In this chapter we give brief details about
- power of attorney
- life insurance
- employment
- help with legal costs
- making a will

All of these can be very complicated. On page 107 we describe where you can get more information and sources of free legal help. See chapter 7 for information on housing law.

Power of attorney

There may be times when a person with AIDS is unable or doesn't want to deal with their financial affairs. One very simple but common problem for carers is not being able to sign cheques on behalf of someone else, for example.

In England and Wales, a Power of Attorney is a document by which one person (the donor) gives another (the attorney) power to act in his or her name. The power may be extremely wide, entitling the attorney to do many things the donor could do – sign cheques, buy and sell investments or property and collect benefits, for example. It can be limited to cover certain areas only.

Power of Attorney can be given only by someone who is capable of understanding what it means. Normally, it will apply only for as long as the donor remains mentally capable of understanding it. If someone becomes very ill or confused this can mean that Power of Attorney is no use when it is most needed. To get round this problem the person with AIDS could set up an *Enduring* Power of Attorney which continues to apply even if this happens. It can be organised so that it comes into effect only in such circumstances. A Power of Attorney *must* be in the form of a deed – signed, sealed and delivered – so you should consult a solicitor unless you are sure how to do it.

In Scotland it is likewise possible for one person to give another the power to act in his or her name, but any power to act stops operating if the donor becomes ill and confused and incapable of understanding it. It is not possible to have an Enduring Power of Attorney in Scotland.

Instead, when someone becomes unable to manage their own affairs, a relative or carer can apply to the Court of Session for the appointment of a *curator bonis* to manage the ill person's affairs under the supervision of the Accountant of Court. The Mental Welfare Commission for Scotland may apply for appointment of a *curator bonis* if no one else does so.

Frontliners (see page 60) have Power of Attorney forms and will provide help.

Some people with HIV suggest giving someone Power of Attorney themselves and are very happy to hand over responsibility to someone they trust. Doing so can be a way of demonstrating this trust and making the relationship a closer one. But it can be very difficult for carers to talk about the possibility of needing Power of Attorney, particularly at times when the person concerned is well.

There is no simple answer to this problem. You may even decide that it might cause too much distress, suspicion or bad feeling to be worth discussing. It may help to talk about how Enduring Power of Attorney might be arranged to apply only in certain circumstances, to act as a kind of insurance policy in case of spells of illness.

The Court of Protection

If someone becomes unable to manage their own financial affairs, and no previous arrangements have been made to cope with this, a carer can apply to the Court of Protection. This gives the person nominated certain rights to use the funds of the person with AIDS for things he or she may need. It is supervised by the Court.

Vesting property

Somewhat simpler and therefore perhaps less threatening than Power of Attorney is vesting property in joint names. This may be particularly appropriate for partners who have no legal relationship with each other.

In the case of money, this may be simply opening a joint bank account. Where housing is concerned, it may involve registering a partner as joint owner – see page 134. Smaller items (such as furniture) can just be given to someone, but if there are likely to be disputes with other people over these, a simple signed and witnessed declaration would be better. Alternatively, specific items can be mentioned in a will, but this won't take effect until after the death of the donor.

There are two advantages to vesting property. The first is that a surviving partner will be able to continue using the property without any problem. Second, there have been cases where a surviving partner of a gay couple has been troubled by relatives who have made unjustified claims on the estate. Relatives may think twice about starting proceedings to upset something which took effect in someone's lifetime, whereas a will might seem easier to challenge. The disadvantage of transferring property into joint names is that it may be difficult to revoke the arrangement if your relationship subsequently turns sour.

Life insurance

No one has a legal right to life insurance or indeed any other kind of insurance. If an insurance company decides that it does not wish to insure someone, that is its own decision, and there is no right to challenge such a decision, no matter how unfair it seems. Nor do you have rights to information about reasons for refusal.

For most people the question of life insurance first arises when trying to get an endowment mortgage. This issue can be avoided altogether. Mortgages do not have to be insured unless the lender requires it. It is usually possible to get a simple repayment mortgage without any sort of life cover.

Insurance contracts are in a special category in that they are said to be of the 'utmost good faith'. This means that if you fail to give information which you know or ought to have known would affect your insurability at the time you completed the proposal form the company can treat the policy as void and refuse to meet any claim. For example, an insurance company could turn down a claim if at the time you completed the proposal you had been diagnosed as being HIV positive, but had not said so.

Insurance companies always ask questions about any recent medical treatment or attention received, and usually ask if any previous application for life insurance has been delayed, refused, postponed or accepted on special terms.

They are now also likely to ask if you have been counselled or medically advised in conjunction with AIDS or any sexually transmitted disease and if you have had a test for HIV. In addition, many now send supplementary questionnaires to single men who apply for life insurance asking if they are gay, bisexual, a drug-user, haemophiliac or the sexual partner of someone in one of these groups. They may also ask if they can approach your doctor for information.

Anyone with HIV is likely to be refused life insurance. Many carers who have not been diagnosed also have problems trying to get insurance. The Association of British Insurers say that you are unlikely to be refused insurance *just* because you have had a test for HIV. However, if an insurance company has good reason to think you are gay or bisexual or have other information they think relevant (about use of drugs or treatment for a sexually transmitted disease, for example), they are likely to refuse insurance – even if you have had an HIV test which proved to be negative.

If you do decide that you would prefer an endowment mortgage, or you require life insurance for any other reason, consider the following:

- Don't be tempted to lie on application forms. If you are found to have been withholding information, either deliberately or unwittingly, a claim may not be paid.
- If you think you may be turned down for life insurance it may be worth using a broker who can give advice about the policies of different companies – the Terrence Higgins Trust and other advice agencies may be able to help (see below).
- If you haven't already had a test for HIV, do not do so until after you have applied for insurance.
- When you apply for life insurance, the proposal form will almost certainly contain a clause stating that you are willing to let the insurance company approach your doctor. If you sign the form you will have given your permission for this to happen. The British Medical Association (BMA) have advised doctors that they must not *speculate* about a patient's lifestyle or about any 'risk' of HIV infection. And a doctor should not comment on your sexuality unless you have given information to the doctor about it. A good doctor should redirect any questions about lifestyle to you anyway, but you may want to think carefully before disclosing such details to your doctor, unless it is necessary for either diagnosis or treatment. Under the Access to Medical Reports Act you have the right both to see reports prepared by your doctor, and to refuse to let the doctor send them.
- If you are asked by an insurance company to have an HIV test, you may decide to refuse, in which case your proposal will probably be turned down. The BMA have issued guidelines to ensure that people who do decide to be tested are properly counselled and are given full information. All doctors who take the blood for an HIV test must counsel you beforehand. After this you have to give consent for the test. The consent form has a space where you can, if you wish, nominate a doctor who will receive the test results if they are positive. The doctor taking the blood for the test will encourage you to do this. You can nominate the doctor, either your own GP or another, who is to perform the test. This doctor will then provide or arrange post-test counselling.

Some insurance companies have life insurance policies which exclude AIDS. The proposal forms do not ask questions relating to HIV, but the policies will not pay out if AIDS was a factor in the death. However, these policies cannot be used as a security for house purchase and there may be problems in claiming because it can be difficult to determine if a death is AIDS-related or not.

THT (page 57) and Immunity (page 107) will give advice and they or your local AIDS helpline may be able to refer you to insurance brokers who may be able to help. In Scotland, ALBA at the Scottish AIDS Monitor will advise on insurance and the law in Scotland – see page 58.

Complaints about insurance companies (such as the pay-out not being what you expected, a claim being refused, or delays) can be made to:

The Insurance Ombudsman Bureau
31 Southampton Row
London WC1B 5HJ   01-242 8613

You can complain only about companies which are members of the scheme (membership is not compulsory). The Ombudsman does not deal with complaints about brokers, or about surrender values of life insurance policies, or about being refused cover in the first place. You should approach the Ombudsman only after you have taken the issue up directly with the insurance company, but within six months of reaching deadlock.

Employment

There are no reported cases of anyone catching an HIV-related illness through normal contact with an infected person at work. In the few occupations where there may be some risk of catching or passing on the virus, such as in the health and emergency services, guidelines have been issued by unions or professional associations which give details of precautions to be taken.

There is therefore no reason to discriminate against people with HIV or their carers at work. Sadly, there have been cases where prejudice from an employer or colleagues has led to a dismissal. In some cases, life has been made so unpleasant that employees have been forced to resign. The stark truth is that it is often very difficult to do anything about this.

Getting a job

The law can neither force you to work for anyone nor force anyone to employ you. An employer can recruit whom he or she likes, as long as there is no discrimination on the grounds of an applicant's sex, race, colour, ethnic origin or marital status. But at present there is nothing to prevent an employer refusing to employ someone on the grounds that he or she has an HIV infection, is a carer, or is someone in what might been seen as a 'high risk group'.

Keeping a job

The law gives some people the right to compensation if they are unfairly dismissed from a job. Cases are heard by an Industrial Tribunal. You have to have been working for your employer for a *qualifying period* of two years (if you work at least sixteen hours a week) or five years (if you work at least eight hours but under sixteen hours a week) before you get this right. This qualifying period does not apply if you have been unlawfully discriminated against because of your sex, marital status or race, or because of your membership or non-membership of a trade union, or because you took part or proposed to take part in certain trade union activities.

People who cannot go to an Industrial Tribunal with a complaint for unfair dismissal include: members of the police service and armed forces; share fishermen; those who normally work outside Great Britain; and those who have reached the normal retiring age for their employment or, if there is no normal retiring age, have reached the age of 65.

A dismissal will be considered to be fair if the employer can show that the reason or principal reason for it was one of a number of specified reasons laid down by Parliament, and the Tribunal is satisfied that the employer conducted a fair investigation and acted reasonably in the circumstances. One reason which could be relevant to HIV is where it is claimed that the dismissal relates to the capability of the employee for doing his or her job.

In cases where an employee is not able to do his or her job or does it less well because of having an HIV-related illness or being a carer, it is likely that a dismissal for this reason would be considered *fair* by an Industrial Tribunal, provided appropriate dismissal procedures had been followed.

The Department of Employment maintains that Tribunals should not take account of any pressure from fellow employees when considering a case. If an employer dismisses someone because of industrial action, or the threat of it, the dismissal *automatically* becomes unfair. Giving way to other kinds of pressure is not automatically considered unfair and some cases have been reported where employers have given in to the prejudices of their staff or customers. Some employers may risk having to pay compensation for unfair dismissal rather than face industrial action or lose a valued customer.

Although this may seem grim, don't assume that there is nothing you can do. Most employers dislike litigation because of the publicity, cost and time involved. It is possible that you can negotiate a compromise. While you may not get your job back, you may get a reference, and some financial compensation.

In cases where an employee's health is deteriorating and he or she is unable to do a job, the Department of Employment recommends that the employer should try to find some other work for him or her. Many carers have to rearrange their working lives to cope with new responsibilities. Your employer may be willing to be flexible and to come to some mutual arrangement with you, although the law does not require them to do this.

Industrial Tribunals

These have been set up throughout England, Wales, Scotland and Northern Ireland. Each Tribunal has three members; one is from the employers' side of industry, one is from the employees' side, and the chairman is a lawyer. The Tribunals have been set up to provide a quick and cheap way of deciding disputes between employers and employees and occasionally between an employee and his or her union.

Industrial Tribunals have a heavy caseload. Only about 30 per cent of cases go all the way to a hearing; most of the others are settled by agreement. Although technically you do not need a solicitor you might find it advisable to have one or get help from another source such as a trade union. Legal Aid will not cover the cost. You can get an application form IT1 (IT1 [Scot] in Scotland) and explanatory booklet ITL1 from your local job centre, most law centres, Citizens Advice Bureaux and local advice centres. To make a complaint, send the completed form to the appropriate Central Office of the Industrial Tribunals:

Central Office of the Industrial Tribunals (England and Wales)
93 Ebury Bridge Road
London SW1W 8RE   01-730 9161

Central Office of the Industrial Tribunals (Scotland)
St Andrew's House
141 West Nile Street
Glasgow G1 2RU   041-331 1601

Central Office of the Industrial Tribunals (Northern Ireland)
16-22 Bedford Street
Belfast
Northern Ireland BT2 7FD   (0232) 327666

When you have made your application, a copy of the form will automatically be sent to the Advisory, Conciliation and Arbitration Service (ACAS) who may try to help you and your employer settle the case privately. The application must be made within three months of the date on which the employment ended.

Constructive dismissal

If you consider you have been forced to resign because of prejudice or discrimination you can still bring a case; the procedure is the same except you will claim for 'constructive dismissal'. You will have to show that your employer behaved in such a way or allowed a situation to develop which was so intolerable that in effect you were forced to leave. However, it is much harder to prove constructive dismissal than unfair dismissal and you will have to show that your employer's conduct was in fundamental breach of contract.

If you win an unfair dismissal case, the compensation you are awarded is subject to a statutory maximum. The amount is based on a *basic award* (maximum £5160 – worked out according to your age, pay and length of service), and a *compensatory award* (maximum £8925 – based on loss of pay, future loss of pay, and loss of statutory rights). If the Tribunal makes an order for reinstatement or re-engagement with which the employer refuses to comply, you may also be entitled to an *additional award* – maximum £4472. The average award in 1987–1988 was £1865.

You will have to pay your costs out of this amount. Although you don't have to use a solicitor to take a case to an Industrial Tribunal, if you do use one you may end up with very little money left over by way of compensation. If you qualify for assistance under the Green or Pink Form Scheme (see below), this should cover a lot of the solicitor's preliminary work, although it will not cover the hearing itself. If you do use the Green Form Scheme there may be a statutory charge on any money received as a result. Some cases are settled beforehand, in which case costs will not be very high.

Wrongful dismissal is not the same as unfair dismissal, although the circumstances of a particular case may give rise to an action for both. A wrongful dismissal occurs when the dismissal amounts to a breach of contract – usually because the employer has failed to give sufficient notice. You may sue for damages in the civil courts – Industrial Tribunals have no power to hear these cases.

An action for wrongful dismissal may still be important if, say, you don't qualify for unfair dismissal because you haven't completed the necessary two years', continuous service. Compensation may be higher as it is based on the actual loss you suffer, on which there is no statutory limit.

Redundancy

You can be made redundant when your employer no longer has enough work for you to do – for example, because a business is closing down, or has changed in some important way.

If you are dismissed because of redundancy it may be possible to claim unfair dismissal if:
- redundancy wasn't the real reason, but was used just as an excuse
- you were unfairly selected for redundancy. You would have a stronger case if your selection did not follow agreed procedures and there was no special reason for ignoring them.

If you are made redundant and you are aged 18 or over, and have been employed in your job continuously for 2 years or more, and have worked at least 16 hours per week, you are entitled to a statutory minimum redundancy payment and a written statement setting out how the payment has been calculated.

More information from Immunity – see page 107.

Help with legal costs

Legal Aid

The Legal Aid system aims to make sure that people can get legal help if they genuinely need it even if they cannot afford the fees. Work for legally aided clients is done by solicitors and barristers (advocates in Scotland) in private practice, and they act in the same way as they would for a fee-paying client, except that their bills are paid out of a government fund.

There are two schemes for civil cases:
- the Legal Advice and Assistance Scheme, otherwise known as the Green Form Scheme (the Pink Form Scheme in Scotland).
- Civil Legal Aid, which covers the cost of making or defending a civil claim – damages for injuries or maintenance on the breakdown of a marriage.

Each scheme has its own detailed rules. Sometimes the help is completely free, sometimes you will have to pay a contribution.

The Legal Advice and Assistance Scheme (the 'Green Form Scheme' in England and Wales the 'Pink Form Scheme' in Scotland)

This scheme is intended to cover help of almost any kind from a solicitor. There are, however, a few limitations:
- It cannot be used to enable the solicitor to appear in court or in a tribunal as an advocate, or to conduct a court case. (However, the solicitor can give preliminary advice and start proceedings.)
- The amount of work cannot usually exceed a cost of £50, unless the solicitor applies to the Legal Aid office for authority to do more.

You apply through your solicitor. He or she will ask you questions about your income, savings and dependants to see whether you qualify, and what contribution you will have to make, if any.

Civil Legal Aid

To get a Legal Aid Certificate you must satisfy a number of conditions:

- you must be financially eligible
- your case must be eligible – claims for libel or slander are excluded
- you must have a reasonably strong case
- it must be reasonable to grant you Legal Aid.

Application is made through your solicitor. You will have to provide basic information about your finances; the DSS will decide if you are eligible or not and will tell the Legal Aid office the maximum contribution you can be asked to pay. It is up to the Legal Aid office to decide if your case *deserves* Legal Aid or not, and what you will be asked to pay. In addition, most solicitors who work for clients under the Legal Aid scheme will give a half-hour's initial advice for £5.

More information·

See the end of this chapter. Also, Lesbian and Gay Employment Rights (LAGER).

> LAGER
> Room 203, Southbank House
> Black Prince Road
> London SE1 7SJ   01-587 1643 (gay men); 01-587 1636 (lesbians)

Making a will

Regardless of the amount of property anybody has at the time of their death, if that person dies intestate (without having made a will), the law will automatically dictate what is to happen. Any property goes to relatives; if you have no relatives, everything goes to the Crown, which means the government gets it.

A will does not just deal with major items of property. It can also include such things as instructions for the funeral and the appointment of guardians for children, as well as being a way of expressing gratitude or friendship by making small gifts. Anyone making a will also has to decide who are going to be the executors – the people responsible for administering their estate (their property and possessions) and looking after their affairs generally.

Many people choose friends or relatives to be executors. Alternatively, a bank manager, solicitor or accountant can be used – in which case their fee will be deducted from the estate. There is no legal requirement that a will should be drawn up or witnessed by a solicitor, and many people draw up their own wills. However, you may consider a solicitor's fee a worth while investment for peace of mind, particularly if the will is likely to be complicated.

The Gay Bereavement Project (see page 262) has long campaigned for partners to make a will if they wish to leave property to each other, They have produced a simple will form which can be used if everything is to be left to the partner. Send an SAE to:

> Gay Bereavement Project
> Unitarian Rooms
> Hoop Lane
> London NW11 8BS

The book *Wills and Probate* (published by Consumers' Association) is a clear guide both to making a will and administering the estate of someone who has died. It costs £7.95 (including p+p). *Make Your Will* and *How to Sort Out Someone's Will* are Action Packs on the same subjects, with several checklists, will forms and other forms as appropriate in the back pocket. They are designed for use only in England and Wales. Each costs £7.95 (including p+p) and is available from Consumers' Association (see appendix).

Immunity (see page 107) has a leaflet on wills, and can give advice.

Nobody has complete freedom to dispose of property in a will. If a dependant or some other *specified* person is cut out of a will, in England and Wales he or she may apply to a Court under the Inheritance (Provision for Family and Dependants) Act 1975. The Act allows the following people to challenge a will on the grounds that it does not make reasonable financial arrangements for them:

- the wife or husband of the person who has died
- a former spouse of the person who has died, who hasn't remarried
- a child of the person who has died
- any person (not being a child of the person who has died) who was treated as being a child of the family
- any other person who was maintained either wholly or partly by the person who has died immediately before he or she died.

The same people can also challenge the way property is distributed under the rules of intestacy. In such cases, it is up to the person alleging that the will was invalid to *prove* the accusation. Judgement would not be given lightly. It might, however, be a good idea to get a doctor to witness the will, just in case.

The Inheritance (Provision for Family and Dependants) Act 1975 does not apply in Scotland, but Scottish law specifies that regardless of what is set out in a will, any widow or widower or any children are entitled to a certain amount of property and/or money from the estate. The law is complicated – see below for where to go for more information.

The most important piece of property which most people will need to consider is their home. Sole owners will need to make their wishes clear in a will. If property is owned jointly the rights of inheritance depend on the type of ownership.

In England and Wales if property is owned by two or more people as 'beneficial joint tenants', each is considered to own the whole property. This means that if one dies, the survivor will automatically own it. These arrangements cannot be altered under the terms of a will. If property is owned by two or more people as 'tenants in common', their respective interests in the property will be quite separate. So, if one dies, his or her share of the property won't automatically pass to the surviving co-owner, but will be distributed under the terms of either the will or the rules of intestacy.

If you are intending to buy a property with someone else, the method of ownership is obviously something to bear in mind and to discuss with your solicitor or licensed conveyancer. If you already own a property jointly and wish to change the type of ownership, you can. It is possible to change a beneficial joint tenancy simply by giving a written notice of your wish to your co-owner(s). You will then be treated as tenants in common.

If, on the other hand, you want to make it clear that you wish to change from holding the property as tenants in common to beneficial joint tenants, so that the survivor(s) will inherit automatically, you should draw up an agreement with your co-owner(s). This will need to state that your intention is to be treated as beneficial joint tenants. You may wish to consult a solicitor to help you with the wording, but this isn't absolutely necessary. The system is different in Scotland – see below for where to get advice.

More information

For more information about legal matters contact the Legal Line at the Terrence Higgins Trust (see page 57), the Advisory Legal Bureau on AIDS (ALBA) – part of the Scottish AIDS Monitor – see page 58), or Immunity (see below). Local AIDS helplines may also be able to give you information or point you to someone who can – a sympathetic solicitor, say. Citizens Advice Bureaux may also help and some have solicitors who hold free advice sessions. If a CAB can't help directly they will usually be able to pass you on to someone else. Most large cities have Law Centres which give free legal advice.

Immunity

Immunity is an organisation which carries out research into HIV. It also has a legal advice centre in London which helps people who have an address in Greater London with legal problems associated with HIV or AIDS. The service is free and wide-ranging – Immunity staff will help take a case to court or tribunal, if necessary. They specialise in the legal side of housing, employment, immigration, insurance, mortgages, wills, family matters and problems relating to medical treatment like consent and confidentiality. All advice is absolutely confidential. You need to phone Immunity to arrange a time to visit.

> Immunity
> 260a Kilburn Lane
> London W10 4BA   01-968 8909

Leaflets are planned on various issues. Titles published so far are as follows. Prices given are for single copies, including postage. *AIDS – the Facts for Working Girls* (written by women prostitutes for women prostitutes) (16p); *HIV, You and the Law* (20p). Your rights in the AIDS era: *Testing* (16p); *Discrimination at Work* (16p); *Your Rights at Work* (16p); *Wills* (16p)

The London Lesbian and Gay Switchboard has a 24-hour phone service which can put you in touch with local solicitors or agencies who will be understanding and sympathetic: 01-837 7324. Gay Legal Advice (GLAD) has gay lawyers who may help: 01-253 2043 (7pm to 10pm, Monday to Friday)

6

Home nursing

The important thing was to give him a cuddle in the morning or whenever it was appropriate

Some people with AIDS have bouts of illness which require intensive nursing at home. This section gives short practical tips on nursing tasks in case you need them. If this looks likely ask the doctor or hospital consultant to arrange for a district nurse or someone from a domiciliary support team to show you what to do. They can demonstrate how, for example, to lift a sick person and how to wash and bathe them. They may also be able to provide any equipment you need.

It is very important not to take over completely if you do hit periods when nursing is required. Although you may have to carry out physical tasks and help the person you are caring for more than usual, it is essential to talk about and agree what you do. You need to find out what the person prefers to do for himself or herself and support and encourage him or her to do as much as possible. This will reduce feelings of dependency, and work against any tendency to become passive. If you feel the person is expecting you to do things he or she is perfectly capable of, you should say so. But be aware of what he or she may be capable of doing – this may vary from day to day. Learn to recognise the signs of real tiredness. Be patient: people who are ill act much more slowly.

When you are about to carry out any nursing task, say what you are going to do. This will allow the person to co-operate, and will prevent any surprises. Don't take unnecessary and offensive precautions against infection. See page 211 for all you need to do. Remember that a very real risk is the person you are caring for catching an infection from *you*.

The environment

The bedroom and other rooms should be changed as little as possible. Remember that anything which has to be done should be for the comfort and benefit of the person you are looking after, not yours. Matters you see as only trifling can be vastly important to a sick person. Slight inconveniences can turn into major frustrations. Try to be aware if any of your own, very reasonable, activities are irritating. For example, the noise made by normal dusting can easily become 'someone banging away with a duster'.

Eating

People who are ill sometimes cannot face food. They may have difficulty swallowing, eating may be painful or their appetite may be affected. You may find that the person you are caring for asks for food but has lost all appetite by the time it has been prepared.

Small helpings and more frequent meals that take little time to prepare may help. Moist, bite-sized food may be more appealing and lots of foods can be pureed or liquidised if there's a problem swallowing. If a sore mouth is a problem, avoid highly spiced, salty or dry foods – soups and liquids help. Using a straw helps when the mouth or tongue is sore, but drinking from a cup may make swallowing easier because raising the head straightens the gullet.

If the person wants to eat only a limited range of foods such as ice-cream and soup you could try food drinks, supplemented with protein and vitamins made up with milk – Complan in various flavours, for example. The important thing is to keep up the intake of fluids to avoid dehydration. Try to encourage this – even small sips of water or sucking an ice-cube will help.

Moving

In lifting anyone, or for that matter any weight, there is one golden rule never to be disregarded – *bend your knees, not your back*. Your knees were designed to fold, while your spine was designed to keep you erect. Try to keep your weight above your feet, and your feet apart for stability. If you have to turn, use your whole body – don't just twist at the waist.

Move slowly and smoothly. This allows you to have more control and will make the person you are helping feel more secure. Practise with a friend – particularly how to cope with someone who falls (see below).

Sitting up in bed

The person should lie on his or her back with bent knees so the feet are flat on the bed. Cradle the shoulders and head with one arm. The person should then push with the feet while you slide the head and shoulders up. Alternatively, you can place both hands under the hips and slide from there. If the person is too weak to assist, you will need someone else to help. Five or six pillows will help someone to rest while sitting up in bed. A footrest or blocks under the two legs at the foot of the bed will prevent him or her slipping down the bed.

Sitting on the edge of the bed

Support the neck and shoulders with one arm, and slide the head and shoulders over to the side of the bed. Move the legs to the same side. Slide an arm under the hips and then pull them towards you so that the person is lying on one side of the bed. Stand beside the bed, one foot in front of the other for support. Bend down and put one arm around the shoulders and the other around the waist. He or she should put one arm round you and push on the bed with the other. Straighten your knees and rock back, pulling the person up with you. He or she should push on the bed, letting the legs slide over the side of the bed. Keep up the support until you are both stable and any dizziness felt by the person has gone.

From a sitting to a standing position
- Be sure that the chair (or whatever) will not tilt or slip.
- The person you are lifting should sit with feet apart and firmly on the floor. Stand with your feet in front to stop him or her sliding forward.
- Bend your knees and place your hands under the armpits (or around the waist – whichever is most stable and comfortable for both of you).
- Keeping your back straight, straighten your knees, so you both come to a standing position.

From a chair or wheelchair to the toilet or to another chair
- Get the person you are helping as close as possible to the toilet or second chair.
- If a wheelchair is involved, make sure the brakes are on, remove the armrest on the side next to the toilet or second chair and lift up the footrest.
- Stand in front.
- Make a sling out of a towel twisted tightly or folded lengthwise. This goes under the person's armpits and around the back.
- Squat down and grip the knees between your own.

- Straighten up, taking the weight in the sling. Pivot on your feet so that the person can swing sideways on to the toilet or second chair. It will help if he or she can clasp hands round your neck.

You can use the same method to help someone move to a chair. Have the chair near to the bed and at about 45 degrees to it. When you are both standing, pivot round and bend your knees so that the person can hold on to the arms of the chair and slide down on to it using your body as support. Remember that someone who has been in bed for a time may be very weak and legs can give way without warning. You should be prepared for this – see below.

Walking
Once you are both standing, the person you are helping should keep an arm round your shoulders. You should put an arm round his or her waist (or take hold of the belt) and help him or her pivot round so you are facing the same direction. Keep on providing support. When the person is steady, begin to walk. You should be providing security and balance, not supporting his or her whole weight.

If the person begins to fall, help by controlling it. Pull him or her towards you. You may be able to lower him or her onto the bed or chair or, if you have been walking, you may both sink to the floor. Let your body act as a slide. Do not try to lower anyone on to the floor while remaining upright as you may hurt your back. Try to use your body as a cushion and to steer away from furniture or other objects. If you are both on the floor you will be able to remain there a while to calm any fears or distress. You will need someone to help get the person back to a bed or chair. In the meantime keep him or her warm with blankets and comfortable with pillows.

Washing and bathing

Skin is living tissue which is continuously being replaced while the old skin dies off and flakes away. It contains sweat glands for controlling body temperature and lubricating the skin. The skin also contains hair, blood vessels to nourish the skin, and nerves which provide information on temperature and pressure. A person who has fevers or night sweats will need bathing frequently to remove the stale sweat and let the glands function more freely. Bathing is also a refreshing relief.

If the skin is dry, don't use soap. Warm water may be enough. If the skin is very dry, pour some bath oil into the water, or use a moisturiser afterwards.

Having a shower is usually easier than a bath. A chair or stool in the shower, as long as it is stable, may help when someone is very weak.

Using a bath
If getting into the bath is difficult, use a special bath board and seat and special rails and handles. These can often be borrowed from social services who may also fit rails and handles if they are needed – see page 54.

- Make sure the bathroom is warm.
- Collect everything that will be needed.
- Run the bath, mix, and test the temperature carefully.
- If the person needs help to get into the bath, stand directly behind him or her, beside the bath.
- The person should clasp his or her hands together in front or grasp one wrist with the other hand. You can then slip your hands under the armpits and grasp the forearms in front of the waist. You should now be providing enough support so that he or she can lift the feet into the bath.
- Bend your knees to lower the person on to the bath board or seat or on to the bottom of the bath.
- To help someone out of the bath, carry out the same operations in reverse order.

Giving a blanket bath
A blanket bath is a 'bath' in bed.

- Make sure the bedroom is warm.
- Collect everything you need, including two flannels (one for the main part of the body, another for the bottom) and an extra towel to put underneath.
- Remove the bed covers, but keep the person warm with a sheet (flannelette is warmer than cotton), large towel or light blanket.
- Slip the extra towel underneath the part you are washing to protect the bed.
- Start with the face, ears and neck. Use a flannel, then rinse and pat dry. Avoid soap on the face in case it gets into the eyes.
- Then wash, rinse and dry each arm from the armpit down to the fingers; followed by chest, abdomen, genital area, back and buttocks. Change the water if necessary.
- Wash each leg, rinse and dry it in the same way that you did the arms. If possible let the person dabble his or her feet in the basin.

- Keep the person covered as much as possible both, to respect modesty and to prevent chilling and make sure that the water does not get cold.
- Be aware of any areas which are specially painful.
- Wear disposable gloves if there is bleeding, faecal soiling or discharge of any sort of body fluid, or if there are lesions or wounds on the skin.

Massage
Massage while washing, and afterwards, helps with the circulation. It also feels good.

Caring for the mouth

The mouth can get very sore and ulcerated and the doctor may prescribe a paint, spray or mouth wash. Frequent applications may be needed. Thrush is also common and requires treatment. Mouth rinses with warm water may be helpful and are essential if the mouth becomes dry and uncomfortable. Don't rinse the mouth if the person is confused and could choke. Don't forget to provide a bowl with a cover to spit into. Cotton buds can be used if a toothbrush causes discomfort. If false teeth are worn ask how they are usually cleaned. Don't forget to rinse them well afterwards.

Caring for the eyes

A healthy person's eyes are kept clean by a fluid that seeps across the eyes automatically. This mechanism doesn't always work when someone is sick and the eyes may need bathing. If so, place a towel around and under the face and, standing behind if possible, swab the eyes by squeezing a few drops of saline solution from a cotton wool swab until both eyes are clean. The saline solution should be 5ml of salt to 600ml of boiled water; if it's difficult to carry out these measurements, water by itself makes a good second best. Always wipe eyes from nose outwards, and use a separate cotton wool swab for each eye.

Shaving

An electric razor is less likely to nick the skin than a blade razor. Take extra care if shaving the person with a blade razor.

Washing the hair

Find a comfortable position that is suitable for a hair wash. The two best positions are sitting up with a basin in front, and lying on the back with the head extending beyond the end of the bed (well supported with towels, for example, under the neck) with a basin on a chair or stool underneath the head. You will need plenty of towels or waterproof sheeting to protect the bedding and floor from splashing.

Clothes

The person you are caring for may want to wear favourite clothes, and wearing something special may become very important. If you can, discourage restrictive clothing. Clothes that can be worn in layers are a good idea as body temperature may change very quickly.

Don't rush the dressing or undressing. It takes much longer to dress or undress somebody else than it does to dress or undress yourself.

- If one arm or leg is weaker than the other, deal with it first when dressing, last when undressing.
- Sleeves can be tiresome, especially if the arm is very weak. Put your own arm in the sleeve from the cuff end. Grasp hands and slide the sleeve on. Then ease the shirt, jacket or whatever round the shoulders until it is in a position for the other arm to be inserted in the same way. The second sleeve is likely to be more difficult than the first but take it gently and remember to pull the garment and not the person.
- Check that there are no uncomfortable wrinkles, that the garment is not tight in one place and loose in another and that the buttons are correct.
- Trousers are easier to put on than sleeves. Both legs can go in more or less simultaneously. Pull each trouser leg on to just above the ankle before pulling it over the rest of the leg. This will prevent it catching on toes or toenails. When both legs are in pull the waist of the trousers up to the person's waist.

Pressure sores

Sitting or lying compresses some part of the body between the bones and the chair or bed. Normally this is of no importance because a healthy person shifts position from time to time, even while sleeping. If through weakness, paralysis, insensitiveness or unconsciousness the person doesn't move the blood supply to the tissue under the point of pressure is cut off. The tissues themselves die and an ulcer is formed. It will show as a red patch, dry or cracking, and can be very painful indeed. The ulcer or pressure sore can grow very rapidly so action should be taken immediately. The most likely parts of the body for a pressure sore to develop are the back of the head, the shoulders, the elbows, the base of the spine, the buttocks, the sides of the hips, the knees and the heels. People who are very thin, unusually heavy or incontinent are most at risk. Dampness on the buttocks, for instance, will greatly increase the possibility of a pressure sore developing there.

Lying on the back is restful and allows a person to change position by rolling over on one side or the other. Lying face down with one or two pillows under the head will avoid pressure on the back or buttocks and may help prevent pressure sores. If moving is difficult, you should regularly help with a change of position every two hours or so. Try to avoid having two skin areas resting on one another. Check that vulnerable skin areas are always dry and clean. Gentle massage may also help, as well as providing comfort and warmth. A moisturising cream will help stop the skin becoming dry and flaky.

There are various devices which may also help. *Ripple mattresses* contain a pump which continuously inflates and deflates different sections of the mattress to alter the points of pressure. *Real or artificial sheepskins, waterbeds and cushions* may also help. For more information, get in touch with your district nurse. If a pressure sore does develop a doctor should be consulted.

Pain control

Some people with AIDS experience periods of pain and there may be times when the person you are caring for feels that he or she just cannot take any more.

Doctors will advise on pain control and may prescribe tablets, suppositories or a course of injections. Pain killers usually have to be taken regularly rather than just at times when the pain is severe. Some people have fears about becoming addicted to pain killers, or about side effects such as drowsiness, nausea, lightheadedness or constipation: the doctor should be consulted about this.

Bed-making

Fresh, clean bed linen will make the person you are caring for feel fresher and cleaner. Change it often. Remove the duvet or bed covers and top sheet. Ask the person in bed to turn on his or her side on the far side of the bed. Roll up the dirty sheet as far as you can towards the back. Tuck one edge of the clean sheet under the mattress and fold the rest concertina fashion close to the patient. Next gently roll the person you are caring for over the clean and dirty sheets to the other side of the bed. Pull the dirty sheet off the bed, and pull the clean sheet over the rest of the bed. A low bed may mean repeated bending for you. If this is likely to cause you strain raise a low bed by putting its feet on four *firm* blocks.

Drawsheets

A *drawsheet* can be made from a piece of material (sheeting or absorbent towelling, for example) about one metre by two. It is placed *across* the bed on top of the bottom sheet. This provides a cool, fresh area which can be renewed without having to remake the whole bed. It is particularly useful if the person has fevers and night sweats. If he or she is sweating regularly a waterproof mattress cover may also be needed to protect the mattress.

When the drawsheet is first put in the bed it should be placed well over to one side. It can then be moved bit by bit, perhaps half a dozen times, before it has to be changed. A clean one can be inserted as the old one is removed. Loose ends should always be pulled taut and tucked in under the mattress.

Bedpans

There may be times when the person finds it difficult to get to the toilet. If using a commode is too difficult, they should use a bedpan or urinal. The bedpan should be warm and dry. If the person you are helping can sit up, even for a short time, things are easier. Be prepared to help with toilet paper if necessary. You should wear disposable gloves. Don't forget a basin of water for washing hands.

Dealing with incontinence

Perhaps one of the most distressing symptoms anyone can have is incontinence, which can affect the bladder, bowels or both. To get over this you have to see it in terms of a practical task which you have to handle as efficiently as possible. Try to be relaxed about it. It is important that you don't give the impression that the task is difficult or distasteful. Make sure there is as much privacy as possible. In time it becomes easier for both of you, and less important. Some people begin to 'leak' without noticing and you have to be tactful about mentioning this or suggesting a waterproof sheet. Cutting down on fluids does *not* usually help. It will help to get advice from your GP or district nurse. Your GP should be able to tell you if there is a *continence adviser* in your area – if you have difficulty finding one, contact:

The Association of Continence Advisers and Incontinence Advisory Service of the Disabled Living Foundation
380–384 Harrow Road
London W9 2HU   01-289 6111

Continence advisers will assess the problem, give treatment where possible and will be able to advise you on dealing with it and on the equipment you may need. The Disabled Living Foundation's publication *Notes on Incontinence* (£2 including p+p from the above address) also gives general help and information about aids and equipment.

You will need special equipment such as pads for the patient to wear and protective covers for the bed. Supplies can be bought from chemists, but you may be able to get them free from the NHS through your district nurse or health visitor. A baby's cot mattress protector makes a good substitute if you can't get a waterproof sheet. Some social services departments have a laundry service for sheets. Sometimes the problem is not lack of control but just not being able to get to the toilet quickly enough. If so, there are various things you can do:

- Buy a commode or bedpan or find out if the Social Services department or British Red Cross Society (see page 75) will be able to lend you one.
- You may be able to make the toilet more accessible – or even get a special one put in – (see page 54).
- If the person you are looking after becomes weak, you can get rails and special seats for the toilet from the Social Services department.

Odour

Despite frequent changes of bedclothes and dressings and frequent bathing some people are conscious of and embarrassed by being smelly. This may be more due to fear than be an actual problem so reassurance may be enough. Otherwise, consult the district nurse or GP who may be able to help with special tablets, appropriate dressings or deodorisers.

Giving a suppository or enema

A suppository is a method of introducing a drug into the body through the rectum. It is made of a substance that melts at body temperature and so can be absorbed. Be warned – it will also melt if held in the hand for long. Don't unwrap a suppository until you are ready to use it. Warm it briefly in the hand before inserting it gently as far as possible. An enema is used to introduce liquid into the rectum, usually to encourage a bowel movement. Enemas usually come complete with a nozzle.

Place a paper towel over plastic sheeting under the bottom. Warm the enema briefly in a jug of warm water. Then break the tip of the nozzle and smear it with petroleum jelly before inserting it gently into the rectum. Squeeze the enema bag so that the contents are squirted into the rectum. Take the nozzle out gently and wrap it in kitchen towel or newspaper for disposal. The person should be encouraged to retain the liquid for as long as possible before having a bowel movement. Insertion of a suppository or an enema is easiest if the person receiving it lies on his or her side. Be sure to explain beforehand what you are going to do, so there is no element of surprise! Wear disposable gloves.

Vomiting

Vomiting should be discussed with the doctor, who may recommend treatment or advise on changes to diet. Have a bowl and mouthwash nearby if there is a likelihood of vomiting. False teeth should be removed if there is time. After you have emptied and washed the bowl leave it nearby in case of another attack. You should wear disposable gloves when cleaning up vomit.

Advice on nursing

Don't be afraid of seeking advice from experts and professionals. Don't be afraid to ask what seem to be 'silly questions'. It is worthwhile making a note of your problems as they arise.

Hygiene

Hygiene precautions are simple:
- Wash your hands before and after carrying out any nursing tasks.
- Check hands for cuts and abrasions and cover with waterproof plaster or dressing.
- Wear disposable latex (rubber) gloves when cleaning up blood, urine or faeces, vomit or any other sort of body fluids. Gloves should also be worn when caring for open skin lesions or wounds, or giving injections.
- You can obtain disposable gloves from chemists. Don't use domestic rubber gloves; surgical gloves are unnecessarily expensive.
- Hot water (60°C), and ordinary detergent are adequate for laundry. A solution of ordinary household bleach (one part bleach diluted with ten parts water) is enough to clean toilets and other soiled surfaces.
- Wear an apron that protects your clothing from shoulders to knees if there is any chance it may get soiled with blood, vomit, urine or faeces.
- Wear a face mask if you are going to be in close proximity with a person with AIDS who is coughing blood or sputum into the air. This is the only time a face mask need be worn.
- Paper and plastic can be put in a plastic dustbin bag. Body fluids and so on should be flushed down the toilet. The toilet, commodes and so on should be cleaned with a disinfectant or bleach solution.
- Needles and syringes (called 'sharps' by nurses) should be sealed in puncture-resistant tins or in a special bin from your hospital or district nurse. Needles should not be recapped or resheathed because of the danger of an accidental prick.

7 Housing

The council put him in bed and breakfast — no cooking facility and he shared a room with three others

Finding accommodation

One of the most serious social problems facing people with HIV illnesses is housing. For many people finding somewhere to live can be an almost insurmountable problem. For those with HIV infection the problems are magnified many times. There is a shortage of housing suitable for people with serious health problems, and people who are ill often have difficulties keeping up their income to pay for accommodation. People with AIDS have also suffered discrimination and harassment. It has been shown that people who are HIV-positive are less likely to develop AIDS if they can maintain a good standard of health. But it is practically impossible to provide any sort of care for someone who has nowhere to live. Being homeless can itself cause and complicate illnesses, through stress, lack of security, not being able to eat properly, being cold or damp and not being able to maintain basic standards of hygiene.

For all these reasons good accommodation is essential. Housing needs to be warm, easy to move around in and easy to manage. It should provide privacy and security – and it needs to be affordable. In this section we outline the main sources of help and information. Note that the *legislation* covering your rights to do with homelessness and being a private tenant is different in Scotland, although your *rights* are similar.

Homelessness

Anyone who is homeless or about to become homeless should contact the local council. But it is a good idea to seek independent advice from an advice centre or a law centre first (see page 107).

Under the Housing Act 1985, local authorities have to find accommodation for homeless people who are in 'priority' need. This includes those who are 'vulnerable' because of ill health or disability, people with dependent children living with them, and pregnant women. People with AIDS who fall into these categories, including those who are experiencing debilitating symptoms, should be covered by this Act. It may be harder to persuade an authority that you are vulnerable if you are HIV-positive and have no other symptoms.

The local authority also has to be convinced that an applicant is really homeless. There are five circumstances which count:

- When the applicant has no legal right to stay in existing accommodation, or a very weak legal right – for example, someone living in temporary accommodation such as a hostel. This includes people who have been or are being threatened with eviction.
- When it is impossible to stay put, despite having a legal right to do so. This covers, for example, people who have been illegally evicted and those who can show that they have been threatened by violence from other residents.
- When it is unreasonable to continue living in existing accommodation. Reasons for this could include the standard of accommodation or cases of harassment by neighbours.
- When existing accommodation does not allow families to live together. Families may include companions and helpers for 'people with disabilities'.
- If someone has no accommodation at all.

Local authorities have no obligation to house someone who has made himself or herself 'intentionally' homeless, although they do have a duty to provide advice and assistance, and ensure that there is temporary accommodation, usually for up to 28 days, while the case is being considered. Very broadly, 'intentional' homelessness means deliberately and knowingly leaving accommodation which is both available and reasonable, or doing something which causes you to have to leave. If the local authority says that someone is not homeless, or that they are intentionally homeless, the person should seek independent advice immediately.

Homeless (but not intentionally homeless) people in priority need can apply to the local authority for help. Whether that authority will have to provide permanent accommodation itself, or will refer the applicant to another authority, will depend on any 'local connection' with the area. This is defined as where a person is 'normally resident' in the area (for six months out of the last 12, or three years out of the last five), is employed there, has a family connection, or other special reasons. If someone needs to be in a particular area because of a course of treatment it is worth suggesting that this qualifies as a local connection. A report on *Housing and HIV Infection*, published by the Local Authority Associations' Officer Working Group on AIDS in December 1988, states clearly that proximity to hospital or care services should be recognised as a local connection.

The local authority must make sure that any qualifying person has accommodation although it does not necessarily have to provide housing itself. The authority may, for example, help with arranging a mortgage or make referrals to other landlords, such as housing associations. This can often take some time. In the meantime the local authority will, if necessary, find temporary accommodation – see below.

Many people with HIV are unwilling to try to obtain housing through the provisions of this Act because they fear that their illness will not be kept confidential. Local authorities may require a lot of personal information, including addresses where applicants have lived in the previous five years and medical information from a hospital or GP.

It is said that some authorities may not be sympathetic and may be unwilling to grant accommodation to anyone with AIDS or even to those they see as being members of a 'high risk group'. Don't be put off by this – local authorities *must* provide or arrange suitable housing for anyone who falls within the scope of the law. The first step is to get in touch with the Council's Homeless Persons' Unit or Emergency Housing Office.

Temporary accommodation

Local authorities often put people in temporary accommodation while considering whether they qualify for permanent housing. Temporary accommodation can range from a bed and breakfast to a hostel or may be in private-leased accommodation which can be better still since it is independent and non-institutional. However, *Housing and HIV Infection* (see above) states that accommodation for people with HIV should have '24-hour access, adequate food storage, preparation and cooking facilities, dry heating, access to laundry facilities and access to private bathing and toilet facilities'. This means that most bed and breakfast places are likely to be unsuitable.

If the local authority does not accept that someone is homeless and they are having to obtain temporary accommodation for themselves, options are likely to be bed and breakfast, hostel or, for those who can afford it, private-leased accommodation. Resettlement units and nightshelters are for people who are homeless and have no money but this sort of accommodation is particularly unsuitable for people with HIV-related illnesses, and should only be an emergency option. These different types of accommodation are described below. For information on what is available in your area, a good place to start is the local housing advice centre – see page 129. Citizens Advice Bureaux may also be able to help.

Resettlement units
These are provided by the DSS to give extremely basic emergency accommodation for people who are completely homeless and have no money. Residents have to pay any charges out of welfare benefits. All resettlement units are supposed to conform to DSS rules but in practice they vary greatly in quality and in the attitudes of their staff. They can be crowded and are sometimes dirty and violent. The units are intended for people who have an unsettled way of life who will ultimately move on into longer-term accommodation.

Nightshelters
This is a loose term for places where homeless people can stay for a few nights if there is nowhere else to go. Nightshelter accommodation is usually offered by the local authority or a charity. Accommodation is likely to be very basic in shared rooms or dormitories. Food is usually provided; some help or advice on accommodation may be given.

Bed and breakfast
Help to pay the rent for bed and breakfast can be obtained by claiming Housing

Benefit from the local council, and Income Support for food and other expenses from Social Security offices. Income Support is paid in arrears so it may be worthwhile applying for a crisis loan from the DSS Social Fund. This can be paid on the day the claimant becomes homeless and is repaid out of benefits (see page 172). Because choice is limited by the amount of benefit available, accommodation is likely to be poor and involve sharing with other people.

Hostels

These may be run by local or national charities, housing associations or by the local authority itself. The length of time anyone can stay in a hostel depends on the individual hostel and can range from one night to a couple of years. Hostels vary considerably in size and facilities; some provide very high quality accommodation while others are extremely poor. Some have dormitory accommodation while others have independent bedsitting rooms. Some provide what is described as 'social care' which can include support from a social worker, counselling and help with claiming benefits. They very rarely offer nursing care. Some cater only for special groups of people such as ex-drug-users or people who have just come out of psychiatric hospital. The cost, up to a national limit, could be paid by the DSS.

Council housing

Most people who are currently diagnosed as having AIDS or who are HIV positive are single people without children. As such, they are less likely to get council housing which is usually allocated on a system which tends to give priority to young families. However, anybody, whether single or not, has rights to housing through local authorities if they are homeless through no fault of their own and in priority need. In most cases this will mean being housed by the council or by a housing association.

Housing associations

Housing associations are non-profit-making organisations which provide low-cost accommodation (mainly rented) for people who are particularly in need. Many associations cater for specific groups, such as elderly people or people with disabilities. A few housing associations have their own waiting lists; most people are nominated for places through local authorities or through referral agencies (eg Citizens Advice Bureaux or local housing advice centres) or are housing association transfers.

Central government provides money for housing associations, which is distributed through the Housing Corporation (Scottish Homes in Scotland). The

Housing Corporation monitors the standard of housing provided by individual housing associations, and has some say in the kind of accommodation they provide. It recognises the need for schemes which cater for AIDS or HIV-related conditions. Housing associations can provide housing with different facilities. The availability of these varies from place to place, from association to association and from time to time. They can include staff to help with domestic tasks, and accommodation with special features (all on one level, easy to manage, for example). To find out more, contact the Housing Advice Centre, if there is one, or the housing or social services department of the local authority. Recently, housing associations which specialise in helping people with HIV have been set up. To find out about latest developments contact your local AIDS helpline. Schemes in existence as we go to press are listed below. For security reasons we give the addresses of the head offices of the organisations concerned. You have to be referred to a housing association by another agency, so don't apply directly to them. So far most are in London. See page 129 for where to go for up-to-date information about what may be available.

Housing projects
The AIDS and housing project

This was set up in 1987 as a pilot project by the Special Needs Housing Advisory Service and the National Federation of Housing Associations. Its main aims are to help housing organisations provide good quality and appropriate accommodation for people with AIDS and HIV-related conditions. It does not provide accommodation itself, but will help any government, local authority or voluntary organisation to do so, by providing information and training.

The AIDS and Housing Project
16–18 Strutton Ground
London SW1P 2HP   01-222 6933

Social Care Resource Centre

In South Wales housing association accommodation is available for people who are HIV-positive. Applicants must be able to show confirmation of diagnosis. To protect confidentiality, addresses will be given only to potential residents.

Social Care Resource Centre
University of Wales College of Cardiff
37 Corbett Road
Cardiff CF1 3EB   (0222) 874000 (x5386)

Hammersmith and Fulham Shared Housing

This organisation provides temporary housing for people with special needs in south-west London by managing properties on behalf of housing associations. They currently have a house in Fulham for men who are HIV-positive or who have ARC or AIDS. This is divided into two fully equipped and furnished flats, each with two bedrooms and designed for two people sharing. Referrals are made by agencies (e.g. social services departments, hospitals, voluntary organisations), who must be able to confirm medical diagnosis.

> Hammersmith and Fulham Shared Housing
> 2nd Floor, Bank Buildings
> Fulham Broadway
> London SW6 1EP   01-381 5412/5367

St John's Housing Association

This housing association provides flats for people with AIDS or ARC. In November 1988 they opened their first complex of six self-contained fully equipped and furnished flats in Paddington. People with AIDS are accepted on a first come first served basis if referred by: the Bishop of London (applications should be sent to Rev T Birchard, 18 Somers Crescent, London W2); Frontliners; Piccadilly Advice Centre; St Mary's or St Stephen's Hospitals; or the Terrence Higgins Trust. People with AIDS must have a severe housing problem and must be physically independent when they move in. Nursing and domestic help are arranged through the statutory services. An emergency nursing service is provided by St Mary's Hospital and staff from St John's are available at any time to sit with residents.

> St John's Housing Association
> 203a Sussex Gardens
> London W2 2RJ   01-724 5840

Strutton Housing Association

This association aims to provide good quality housing for anyone who is HIV positive or who has AIDS. They do this by managing housing projects on behalf of other organisations. So far, they have thirteen flats (in Brent, Hackney and Haringey) but hope to have at least 30 by April 1990. Referrals are taken in rotation from the British Refugee Council, Frontliners, the London, Middlesex, St Mary's and St Stephen's Hospitals, Piccadilly Advice Centre, Threshold Housing Advice Centre (in Hammersmith and Wandsworth) and the Terrence Higgins Trust.

Accommodation is in self-contained one-or two-bedroom flats which are designed to make it easy for people to take care of themselves. Partners and carers can stay with a person with AIDS, although they will not have security of tenure if the person with AIDS dies. If necessary, staff can assist in getting practical services such as home helps, Meals on Wheels and nursing care.

> Strutton Housing Association
> 8 Strutton Ground
> London SW1P 2HP   01-222 5921

Other accommodation
St Mungo FLAGs

The St Mungo FLAGs (Family Life AIDS Groups), part of the St Mungo Community Trust, set up their first 'family home' for people with AIDS in Fulham. It is intended for people who have AIDS but are in a state of remission, and who would otherwise have to stay in hospital or bed and breakfast accommodation because they have nowhere else to go. Accommodation is for people who do not feel able to live on their own and prefer living with others in a group or 'family' setting. People are encouraged to be as independent as possible, but domiciliary and nursing support can be arranged. Referrals are taken only from St Stephen's Hospital.

The house can accommodate three people, who share it with a resident carer. There is also a guest flat where visitors can stay for short periods. The DSS pay bed and breakfast charges for residents. The Riverside Health Authority funds a worker to provide assistance and to set up more family homes.

> The St Mungo Community Trust
> Bishop Creighton House
> 378 Lillie Road
> London SW6 7PL   01-381 6680

Cave House

Cave House provides residential accommodation for people with AIDS or ARC. It offers long-term accommodation, including support towards the end of an illness, as well as respite or temporary hospitality. Accommodation is in six flatlets, each with its own kitchen. Three paid staff and volunteers provide help, but the management of the home is the responsibility of residents. Referrals are taken from major AIDS hospitals in London and from social services.

Cave House
PO Box 242
London SE26 5ED

Trans Pennine Housing
Consortium (TPHC)

TPHC work within the boundaries of the regional health authorities of Mersey, Northern, North West, Trent and Yorkshire. They are composed of a consortium of voluntary groups concerned with HIV, housing providers and other specialist agencies. They have an increasing number of houses and flats for single people or families. They also work with local authorities to find emergency accommodation for people who are homeless or in stressful situations. They will give advice about housing, entitlement to welfare benefits and possible source of financial support; they can also help with applications for grants.

Trans Pennine Housing Consortium
St Margaret's Chambers
5 Newton Street
Manchester M1 1HE   061-236 6332

**Where to go for more
information about Housing**
In London:

Frontliners can refer people with AIDS or ARC to suitable housing associations – page 60. Body Positive can refer people with HIV to suitable housing associations – page 59. THT can help with legal advice and also make referrals to suitable housing associations – page 57. Immunity can help with legal advice – page 107. You may also be able to get help from local London HIV groups or Borough HIV offices. Advice centres that can give information about HIV-related housing issues are: Piccadilly Advice Centre   01-434 3773

SHAC (The London Housing Aid Centre)
For families in London only.
189a Old Brompton Road
London SW5 0AR   01-373 7276

Housing Advice Switchboard
For single people and people without children. 01-434 2522 (10am to 6pm, Monday to Friday, general and emergency advice);
(6pm to 10am every day, emergency advice only).

Threshold Housing Advice Centre
126 Uxbridge Road, London W12 8AA   01-749 2925

101a Tooting High Street
London SW17 0SU   01-682 0322

The Angel Project (Inner City Action on Drugs)
Can help with housing issues for drug users
38 Liverpool Road
London N1 0PU   01-226 3113

Outside London

Much less help may be available in other parts of the country. Shelter (National Campaign for the Homeless) manage or fund a number of Housing Aid Centres throughout the country. For details of the nearest contact:

01-253 0202 (England)
031-226 6347 (Scotland)
(0792) 469400 (Wales)

Help is often available from local AIDS helplines or Borough Council offices. Help may also be available nationwide from Frontliners (page 60). Legal help with housing problems is available from the THT (page 57) and Immunity (page 107).

Lothian Regional Council's Supported Accommodation Team AIDS (part of Social Work Department) deals with accommodation for people with HIV or AIDS. It aims to find accommodation in ordinary housing and provide visiting support to residents: 031-556 9140

Some other local authorities also have supported accommodation schemes. These may be single or shared tenancies in local authority or health authority accommodation. Support and advice on housing issues may also be available and support workers may offer to help negotiate changes or improvements. Contact your local authority.

General

Some local authorities have a housing advice centre. Citizens Advice Bureaux also give advice on housing.

Housing law

Some people with HIV have had problems with landlords. The law relating to landlord and tenant is extremely complicated and if you are experiencing problems and are in any doubt about your rights, you should seek advice immediately from a Citizens Advice Bureau, local authority advice centre, one of the housing advice centres listed on page 129 or a solicitor. A brief outline of some considerations is given below.

Private tenants

The rights of private tenants depend on what kind of tenancy or licence they have. Until January 1989, the majority of residential lettings by private landlords were regulated tenancies under the Rent Act 1977 (as amended). After the 1988 Housing Act, which came into force for private tenants on 15 January 1989, tenancies will generally be either assured tenancies or assured shorthold tenancies. It is important to find out what kind of tenancy you have so that you know what your rights are if the landlord wants to evict you, and what you can do if the rent goes up too much.

Shared accommodation

If you share accommodation with your landlord (i.e. share such things as a kitchen, toilet or bathroom, *not* just communal facilities such as a front door or stairway) you have very few rights. Since the new Housing Act such landlords can evict tenants without going to court. Tenants whose agreement began before this cannot be evicted without the landlord going to court, although the courts will always give the landlord of shared accommodation possession. If you have a tenancy which dates from before the new Act and you agree to a change of rent you will be considered to have a new agreement and your landlord can evict you without going to court.

Regulated tenancy

Those who were renting their home before the new Housing Act came into force are likely to have a regulated tenancy if the landlord lives in another building or in another part of a purpose-built block of flats. A regulated tenancy gives a tenant the protection of fair rent and security of tenure.

- The landlord, tenant or both can apply to the rent officer for a fair rent to be registered.

- If the tenancy is not for a fixed term the tenant is entitled to a notice to quit. The landlord (whether the tenancy is for a fixed term or not) cannot regain possession of the accommodation without a court order.

An order for possession will be made only if the landlord can establish one of the grounds for possession set out in the Rent Act 1977. Some grounds for possession are mandatory (the court has to give landlords possession of the property) – an owner returning to live in his home, for example; others are discretionary (it is up to the court to decide what remedy to adopt). These include cases where rent has not been paid, or where tenants have created a 'nuisance', for example.

Being HIV-positive, a person with AIDS or gay are not grounds that are recognised under the Rent Act and no one can be legally evicted for these reasons. If there is any doubt whether or not a regulated tenancy exists either the landlord or the tenant may apply to the county court for a decision.

Assured tenancy

Anyone who moved into their home after 15 January 1989 who has exclusive use of at least one room, and whose landlord doesn't live in the same house, is likely to be an assured tenant unless they have signed an assured *shorthold* tenancy agreement (see below).

- Rent will be agreed by the landlord and tenant and this will be a 'market' rent. The agreement may contain a rent review mechanism; if not, the landlord may propose a rent increase by serving notice on the tenant. The tenant may refer this to the Rent Assessment Committee for consideration. The Committee will fix what it thinks the market rent for the property should be. However, if the landlord and tenant want to come to some other agreement about the rent, they may do so.
- The tenant is entitled to a period of notice to quit and the landlord cannot regain possession without a court order.

The new Housing Act 1988 has brought in some grounds for possession which did not exist before, some of which are mandatory and some discretionary. One of the new mandatory grounds is where more than three months' rent is outstanding. If you have problems paying rent, you should get advice immediately. As before, being HIV-positive, a person with AIDS or gay are not grounds recognised under the Housing Act and no one can be legally evicted for these reasons.

Assured shorthold tenancy

An assured shorthold tenancy is a tenancy which has been granted for an initial fixed period of at least six months. The written agreement has to be in a particular form to be valid. The tenant has no rights to renewal. However, if at the end of the initial fixed period the tenant continues to live in the accommodation the assured tenancy persists if the landlord continues to accept rent.

- The tenant can apply to the Rent Assessment Committee for a determination of the rent at the start of the initial fixed period. Unlike an assured tenancy, the rent that is assessed will be the maximum that can be legally charged by the landlord.
- Grounds for possession, and procedure of giving notice to quit followed by going to court, applies as for an assured tenancy. However, if the term of the tenancy is at an end, and the landlord has given at least two months' notice, he/she will automatically be granted possession by the court.

Licences

Until the introduction of the 1988 Housing Act, many landlords used written licence agreements to avoid establishing a regulated tenancy. This is likely to diminish with the introduction of assured shorthold tenancies since automatic possession, after the fixed period of the tenancy, is guaranteed. People with sham licence agreements may well be regulated tenants if they moved in before 15 January 1989, and it's important to get legal advice about this before signing any new agreement. It is possible that people who live in bed and breakfast accommodation could be assured tenants as receiving board no longer prevents someone being a tenant.

Problems with landlords
Illegal eviction

Most tenants cannot be evicted without the landlord going to court first. This applies to council tenants, regulated tenants, assured tenants and assured shorthold tenants. It does not apply to tenants who share living accommodation with their landlord and moved in after 15 January 1989. Some licensees have also been excluded from protection as a result of the Housing Act.

It is a criminal offence for a landlord to evict a tenant without going to court first. It is also a criminal offence, known as *harassment*, for a landlord to do anything knowing that it is likely to cause a tenant to give up his or her home. Threats and verbal abuse are obvious examples of harassment, and so is not paying the gas or electricity bill so that they get cut off. Illegal eviction and harassment are offences for which there is a current maximum penalty of an unlimited fine and/or two years' imprisonment. Tenants who have been illegally evicted or forced out of their home by harassment can claim damages from their ex-landlord. Tenants who have been illegally evicted, or who are being harassed by the landlord, should seek advice from the council's Tenancy Relation Officer (if there is one), Housing Aid Centre or an independent advice centre such as a Citizens Advice Bureau. In cases of harassment it is important to keep a record of what happens and, if possible, get a witness of the harassment, as the case may go to court.

Inheriting a tenancy

You may have the right to continue living in the property when the tenant dies if you are the tenant's spouse or somebody living with the tenant as his or her husband or wife (common-law husband or wife), or another member of the tenant's family, providing the house or flat was your principal home at the time of the tenant's death. It is unclear whether 'common-law' husband or wife covers gay partners, therefore you should seek advice from a law centre.

Rights of succession for regulated tenants have been amended by the new Housing Act. If the tenant of a regulated tenancy dies, only his or her spouse (or common-law husband or wife) can succeed to the tenancy on the same terms as before. Family members can succeed to the tenancy only if they have lived with the tenant for at least two years before his or her death. The tenancy succeeded to will be an assured tenancy not a regulated one. If the tenant of an assured tenancy dies, then his or her spouse (or common-law husband or wife) is the only person who can succeed to the tenancy. There is no succession to assured shorthold tenancies.

It may be a good idea to take out a tenancy in joint names in the first place. This would give you both equal rights to stay in your home if the other died. The disadvantage of a joint tenancy is that each tenant is jointly liable for the acts and omissions of the other. The landlord may agree to convert an existing sole tenancy to a joint one although he or she is not obliged to do so.

Home owners
Difficulties paying a mortgage

If someone becomes too ill to work, and qualifies for income support, the DSS can give financial help to cover the interest payments on a mortgage, and for ground rent – see page 168 for details. You cannot get DSS help towards paying the capital repayments. How much of the mortgage DSS payments will cover depends on the type of mortgage and the number of years it has been in existence. For example, payments made during the first few years of a repayment mortgage are nearly all interest payments, and so will be covered almost entirely; later on a greater proportion of the mortgage goes to pay off the capital borrowed.

If keeping up payments becomes difficult, it is important to inform the lender about the problem before it gets out of hand. Lenders can be reluctant to take action against borrowers and it may be possible to come to some agreement which will enable the person to stay in the property. However, as a last resort, the lender has the right to sell the property. It has to be sold vacant, and the lender will be able to get a court order to evict if necessary. The court can delay giving the lender this order so it is worth appealing. If the property is sold, the lender is entitled only to the money owing to him and any balance will be paid to the borrower. The lender has to make reasonable attempts to get a good price.

Adaptations

A badly designed or badly equipped home can mean that getting certain things done is unnecessarily difficult. The occupational therapist at your social services department should be able to advise on alterations which may solve these problems. 'Adaptations' means any equipment which is fixed, large or small. These include non-structural fixtures and fittings such as rails, hoists and even structural modifications such as a downstairs toilet. Various grants and allowances are available to help with the cost of installing special facilities. Some you get as a right if you meet certain conditions, while others depend on the policy of your local council. Don't be put off by other people's experiences; councils may do more for people who have pressing needs than they will for others.

Council tenants – the housing department of the local authority is responsible for structural modifications made to accommodation owned or managed by them. They can be approached directly or through the social services department.

Housing association tenants – for structural modifications go to the housing association, otherwise to the social services.

Home owners and people who rent from private landlords – talk to the social services department first. They will tell you what help you can get locally – this may be a grant from the social services, or they may even make arrangements to have the adaptation or improvement carried out. Otherwise, talk to the home improvements officer at your local council about applying for an *intermediate* or *improvement grant* (*standard* grant in Scotland). You have to pay for part of the cost; the actual proportion will vary depending on the type of work proposed and your financial means. If you are a tenant you have to get your landlord's permission first. A completely new system of renovation grants, including grants to help disabled people, is expected to come into operation in April 1990 – check the position with your council.

More information on adaptations can be obtained from: *Housing Booklet No 14: A Guide to Home Improvement Grants* from your library, Citizens Advice Bureau, town hall or Department of the Environment, Room N12/12, 2 Marsham Street, London SW1P 3EB.

8

Transport

Transport can be a problem for anyone who is ill. Using public transport may involve long walks to bus stops or stations and lengthy periods of waiting, and there are sometimes difficulties dealing with crowds and other discomforts. Some people, particularly if they become self-conscious about their appearance, are uneasy about going out generally.

Below we give details of the financial help and practical assistance available for people who find using public transport difficult, and details of help you can get with taxi fares and special transport services. On page 154 we give details of parking and other concessions for drivers.

A comprehensive summary of all these can be found in *Door to Door*, published by the Department of Transport, which is available through local authorities, social service departments, voluntary organisations, libraries and Citizens Advice Bureaux. It is also on sale (price £2.50) from HMSO and other bookshops.

Local transport

Buses and Underground
Most local authorities have schemes which offer 'people with disabilities' reduced or free transport on local buses and, in cities which have them, underground railways. Who qualifies for these varies from area to area.

Some bus companies now have special transport schemes which make it easier for people who would have difficulty using a normal bus. These may consist of adapted buses running on normal routes or special buses which may deviate from a route to pick you up. A few bus operators have schemes in which volunteers are available to help people on and off buses.

Travelling on the London Underground almost always involves some stairs. Details are given in *Access to the Underground: a Guide for Elderly and Disabled People* from the Unit for Disabled Passengers at London Regional Transport. LRT will also do all they can to help people who might have difficulty using the underground:

> London Regional Transport
> 55 Broadway
> London SW1H OBD   01-222 5600

The Docklands Light Railway and the Tyne and Wear Metro are fully accessible, including for those who use wheelchairs. The Glasgow Underground is not accessible to wheelchair users, but facilities for other people with mobility difficulties are good. The Merseyrail Underground has lifts at some stations and access is being improved at others.

You should be able to get information about concessionary fares and special services from your local transport authority or company – look under their name, under Bus and Coach Services in the Yellow Pages or in the 'Community' pages of a Thomson local directory.

Dial-a-ride

There are now about 120 *Dial-a-ride* or *Ring and Ride* services in the UK. Although organised in different ways, they all aim to transport people door-to-door within a certain area. The service can be used for all kinds of social trips but not usually for hospital appointments or going to work. Vehicles are adapted to make them very easy to get in and out of, and nearly all of them can accommodate wheelchairs. The driver will be specially trained in helping people in and out. Bookings are usually made by telephone. Fares are usually low, and often pegged to the cost of travelling by bus. Users usually have to register with the service before using it; all dial-a-rides allow them to travel with a companion.

The social services, Citizens Advice Bureau or local transport department should know of any dial-a-ride services in your area. Otherwise contact:

National Advisory Unit
Keymer Street
Beswick
Manchester M11 3FY   061-273 6038

London Dial-a-Ride Users'
  Association
25 Leighton Road
London NW5 2QD   01-482 2325

Taxis

People with ARC or AIDS may be eligible for a local concessionary fare scheme using local taxis. See page 154 for details of the London taxicard scheme which enables cardholders (and a companion) to travel by taxi for £1 for most journeys. Outside London your social service department should have details of any scheme operating in your area. Some areas have shared taxi or hire car schemes; journeys are booked in advance and the cost is shared between passengers – you don't all have to be picked up or get off at the same place. Contact the social services department or transport department at your local authority for information. Some cities (including London) and towns now have wheelchair-accessible taxis.

Help from volunteers

Many local voluntary organisations (such as WRVS, British Red Cross, St John Ambulance, Lions and Rotary Clubs) have special transport schemes using volunteer drivers. Journeys can be for any purpose – the British Red Cross in particular has a particularly comprehensive service. The St John Ambulance can arrange transport to and from hospital and plans to provide transport for other purposes such as visiting relatives or shopping. Their Medical Department, with the Automobile Association, can arrange transport home for people who are taken ill abroad. Local branches are listed in the phone book.

National Headquarters
St John Ambulance
1 Grosvenor Crescent
London SW1X 7EG   01-235 5231

In addition there may be a community transport scheme offering a similar service or there may be an ambulance or van which can be used to ferry people around by request. To find out what exists locally get in touch with your local Council for Voluntary Services – see page 74.

Social services
Social services departments (social work departments in Scotland) provide transport for people with mobility difficulties to and from some services provided by the department. Transport is usually in groups. Vehicles may be available at other times for essential journeys and, in some areas, volunteer drivers will help with shopping and other essential journeys.

Hospital and ambulance services
The local ambulance service will take people to and from hospital at the request of a GP. Transport may be by car or ambulance depending on the person's needs and what vehicles are available. See also page 75 for details of transport arranged by the British Red Cross.

Longer journeys

Help is available from most long-distance transport operators, although this usually means that arrangements have to be made in advance.

Journeys by air
If special help or facilities are needed, tell the travel agent or airline when you book – an INCAD (Incapacitated Passengers Handling Advice) form has to be filled in. You may be able to fill this in without revealing the nature of the diagnosis, but contact the THT (page 57) for advice first. Airlines have a legal duty to tell the port health authority at the destination about any passenger who has an 'infectious disease' – it is possible that an airline may consider that this applies to AIDS too.

Help will then be waiting both at the airport and in the plane. There is generally no problem about wheelchairs although no one is allowed to sit in one during the flight. Toilet facilities can cause difficulties – if assistance is needed the airline might not let the passenger travel without a companion who can help. Most planes on long-haul flights do have special toilets – check with the airline. Travel-Care provide help at both Gatwick and Heathrow airports and for transit passengers. This can include escorts to the plane, wheelchairs, support and counselling (by qualified social workers) or even just somewhere quiet to sit.

> Heathrow Travel-Care
> Room 1214, Queens Building
> Heathrow Airport TW6 1JH
> 01-745 7495 (9am to 6pm, Monday to Friday; 9.30am to 4.30pm, weekends)

Gatwick Travel–Care
Gatwick Airport
West Sussex RH6 ONP
(0293) 504283 (9.30am to 5.30pm, Monday to Friday; 9.30am to 4.30pm, weekends)

More information is given in *Door to Door* (see above), *Care in the Air — Advice for Handicapped Travellers* from:

Air Transport Users' Committee
2nd Floor, Kingsway House
103 Kingsway
London WC2B 6QX   01-242 3882

Directory of Airline Facilities for Disabled People is available from RADAR (see below); it costs 60p (including p+p).

Incapacitated Passengers Air Travel Guide is free from:

IATA
Publications Assistant
PO Box 160
1216 Geneva
Switzerland

Journeys by train

For details of cheaper fares, see page 154. Any other people who are entitled to Attendance, Mobility or Severe Disablement Allowance or who are registered blind or partially sighted can apply for a Disabled Person's Railcard which entitles the holder and a companion to reduced fares.

InterCity trains have space for a wheelchair, as long as it is no wider than 670mm (26.5 inches). In some others a wheelchair can be manoeuvred inside but once there the passenger has to transfer to a seat. Some InterCity trains have wheelchair-accessible toilets. Some local and cross-country trains have sliding doors and low floors and enough space for a wheelchair to stand between the doors. You will need to check that the stations you want to use are accessible. If you tell the manager of the station you are leaving from, he or she will make sure any help you need is waiting for you. This can include assistance from BR staff, a wheelchair to take you to the train, or whatever else is needed to make the journey possible. Try to give at least two days' notice with details of the help needed.

More information in the leaflet *British Rail and Disabled Travellers* and *Disabled Person's Railcard* from your railway station or Citizens Advice Bureau.

Special toilets

Anyone in a wheelchair knows that journeys are largely planned according to the location of accessible toilets. RADAR publish a list of these and will send it with a special key (they are all locked) if you send £3.25 to:

RADAR
25 Mortimer Street
London W1N 8AB   01-637 5400

Planning journeys

Tripscope provide information to help people plan journeys, using any special facilities or assistance that may be needed. They will also tell you about travel facilities and assistance available in your area as well as helping with longer trips. Free information is given by phone or by letter:

Tripscope
63 Esmond Road
London W4 1JE   01-994 9294 (9.30am to 5pm, weekdays)

9

Cash help

Social security and other benefits

This section describes the main social security and other benefits people with AIDS and carers can claim. It's not an easy read because there are some 50 benefits and concessions which may be relevant, and they each have different rules about who is eligible for them.

Below, we describe the main benefits people can get in several situations – off work through illness, spending time looking after someone, having problems with transport, for example. If you find this heavy going, you can get general advice or information about the whole range of social security benefits from the Department of Social Security (DSS) freephone enquiry service – dial (0800) 666555 for England, Scotland and Wales; (0800) 616757 in Northern Ireland. The service does not have access to personal papers. Each Citizens Advice Bureau has a welfare rights specialist who will be able to help. If they can't answer your questions directly they have a special arrangement whereby they can get advice by consulting the Welfare Rights Service of the THT (page 57). You can also ask the THT yourself, and SAM (page 58) and Immunity (page 107) can also give advice. See page 176 for details of grants and loans from private funds and charities. Your local AIDS helpline may also be able to assist. Some local authorities have a welfare rights officer who may also be able to help. It is essential to get independent advice before you apply. But once you are armed with enough information and are able to argue your case get in touch with your local social security office as soon as possible.

Individual benefits are described in various leaflets; we give references in the text, and there is a list of more general guides on pages 145–6.

For complicated cases the Disablement Income Group has an advisory service.

Disablement Income Group
Millmead Business Centre
Millmead Road
London N17 9QU   01-801 8013

Apart from a special fund set up to help people with haemophilia and HIV, there are no specific benefits for people with AIDS, ARC or HIV infection. However, you will be entitled to the benefits for people who are ill, off work or who have disabilities. Don't be put off by the names of these benefits or because they seem to apply mostly to people in different situations to you.

Many claims for benefits which you can get because you are ill or disabled need a doctor's signature or name and address. But it doesn't have to be your GP: a doctor who knows you at a clinic or hospital will do equally well. Make sure that the doctor's diagnosis is back dated to the earliest possible date because of the 28-week delay in claiming some benefits.

Confidentiality

Confidentiality is important, not least because of the prejudice and stigma which still surrounds AIDS. Sadly, confidentiality is not always maintained. Many people have not claimed benefits because of their fears that confidences would not be respected. It is not necessary to mentioned HIV or AIDS on some documents, but your doctor may want to do so. You can ask your clinic or hospital doctor to carry out any necessary paperwork rather than your GP if you feel that he or she won't co-operate. Also, a consultant's opinion may carry more weight with the Department of Social Security.

In this chapter we describe the benefits for several different situations.

UNEMPLOYED
    Unemployment Benefit   page 147

YOU HAVE TO TAKE TIME OFF WORK BECAUSE YOU ARE ILL
    Statutory Sick Pay   page 148
    Occupational Sick Pay   page 149
    Sickness Benefit   page 149

YOU ARE NOT ABLE TO WORK BECAUSE YOU ARE ILL – AFTER 28 WEEKS
    Invalidity Benefit   page 150
    Severe Disablement Allowance   page 151

YOU ARE UNLIKELY EVER TO BE ABLE TO RETURN TO WORK
    Incapacity Pension   page 153

YOU HAVE DIFFICULTY GETTING ABOUT
    Mobility Allowance   page 153
    Other help with transport   page 154

YOU ARE BLIND OR PARTIALLY SIGHTED   page 155

YOU NEED SOMEONE AROUND TO HELP
    Attendance Allowance   page 155
    Independent Living Fund   page 156
    Severe Disability Premium   page 157

YOU ARE LOOKING AFTER SOMEONE
    Invalid Care Allowance   page 157

WHEN SOMEONE DIES
    Funeral expenses   page 158
    If you are widowed   page 158

MATERNITY AND CHILDREN

Statutory Maternity Pay   page 160
Maternity Allowance   page 160
Free prescriptions and dental treatment   page 160
Maternity Payment   page 161
Child Benefit   page 161
One Parent Benefit   page 161
Additional Tax Allowance   page 161

YOUR CHILD IS SERIOUSLY ILL OR DISABLED page 162

YOU HAVE HAEMOPHILIA page 162

YOU WERE INFECTED AT WORK page 163

YOU WERE INJURED BY CRIME page 163

YOU GO INTO RESIDENTIAL CARE, A NURSING HOME OR HOSPICE page 163

MONEY OFF YOUR RATES page 164

YOU HAVE A LOW INCOME

Income Support   page 165
Housing Benefit   page 166
Family Credit   page 169
Free NHS Charges   page 169
Money from the Social Fund   page 170

Remember that as soon as your income drops because you are out of work or ill, you can apply for the means-tested benefits – Income Support and Housing Benefit. If you're on a low wage and have a family, you can also claim means-tested benefit, Family Credit.

All earnings and benefits are given as weekly amounts unless we say otherwise. Social security benefits are correct for the year beginning April 1990 but most will go up each April – see page 172 for details of how to find out the current rate. Details of taxation are correct for the year beginning April 1989

All claims should be made to your local social security office, unless we say otherwise.

UNEMPLOYED
YOU ARE UNEMPLOYED THROUGH NO FAULT OF YOUR OWN
(see general booklet FB.9 'Unemployed?')

Unemployment Benefit (UB)

Details
£37.35 taxable, for up to 12 months. Spells of unemployment with eight weeks or less between them count towards the 12 months. Depends on your having paid sufficient NI contributions, and you have to be 'actively seeking work'. Sign on on your first day off work, as Unemployment Benefit cannot be backdated.

Additions for dependants?
£23.05 for a dependent adult* if he/she is earning less than this. Nothing for children.

Other notes
If you become ill while unemployed, send a 'Doctor's Statement' to your Unemployment Benefit office and claim Sickness Benefit instead (see below). You can also claim Income Support (see page 165) to top up Unemployment Benefit, or if you are not eligible for Unemployment Benefit.

How to claim
Take your NI Numbercard and P.45 form (which your last employer should have given you) to your local Unemployment Benefit office and fill in a claim form. If you are under 18, take them to your local Careers office. You should also register for work at your local Job Centre.

More information
Leaflet NI.12 'Unemployment Benefit'

---

* A dependent adult is your husband or wife; or another person living with you and looking after your children.

YOU HAVE TO TAKE TIME OFF WORK BECAUSE YOU ARE ILL
(see general booklet FB.28 'Sick or disabled?')

YOU WORK FOR AN EMPLOYER

Statutory Sick Pay (SSP)

Details
£52.50 if you are earning £125.00 or more, £39.25 if you are earning between £46.00 and £124.99. Paid for up to 28 weeks. This is a Social Security benefit but is paid by your employer after deduction of tax and NI. If you take spells off work with eight weeks or less in between them, these will all count towards your 28 weeks. Only spells of sickness lasting 4 or more days in a row count for SSP.

Affected by periods in hospital?
No

Additions for dependants?
No

How to claim
Tell your employer you are ill, and after seven working days send in a 'Doctor's Statement'. Employers may ask you to fill a self certificate for the first 7 days of sickness.

The 'Doctors Statement' does not have to give the cause of the illness. Whether it does so will be up to the doctor so you should talk to him or her first. Change doctors if necessary. If the employer does not accept the evidence of the note you can ask for a formal decision to be given by the independent Ajudication Officer based at the local DSS. This may involve seeing a doctor in the Regional Medical Service. This doctor may discover that the illness relates to HIV but this information is not passed on to the employer or anyone else – he or she is bound by medical ethics and DSS guidelines.

Some people have to take frequent short spells off work. When someone has had at least four self-certificated sicknesses in a year, and the employer isn't convinced the illnesses are genuine, the employee may be asked to see a company doctor for confirmation. An employer cannot compel anyone to do this but may refer the case to the DSS if there are still doubts. The DSS will ask the employee to see his or her own doctor the next time he or she is sick, and the doctor will be asked to give a medical report to a doctor in the Regional Medical Service. This can be done only with the employee's consent. The RMS will be asked for an independent medical opinion and, based on this, the Adjudication Officer at the DSS will decide whether the employee is fit for work. The employer is told of the decision, but *NOT* given any medical details or information which would indicate that an HIV-related illness was involved.

More information
Leaflet NI.244 'Statutory Sick Pay – check your rights'

Occupational Sick Pay (OSP)

Details
OSP is paid by many employers as well as SSP. The amount paid, and the length of time it is paid for, varies from employer to employer and sometimes depends on how long you have worked for the firm.

More information
Ask your employer for details.

YOU ARE SELF-EMPLOYED AND HAVE PAID SUFFICIENT NI CON-TRIBUTIONS
or
YOU ARE UNEMPLOYED AND ILL
or
YOU ARE EMPLOYED BUT NOT ENTITLED TO STATUTORY SICK PAY

Sickness Benefit (SB)

Details
£35.70, tax-free for up to 28 weeks. If you take spells off work with eight weeks or less in between them, these will all count towards your 28 weeks, and you will then qualify for Invalidity Benefit.

Additions for dependants?
£22.10, taxable, for a dependent adult (A dependent adult is your husband or wife; or another person living with you and looking after your children.) if he or she is earning less than this; nothing for children.

Affected by periods in hospital?
Reduced by £18.80 after 6 weeks in hospital, or by £9.40 if you have a dependant.

Other notes
With the agreement of a doctor and the local Social Security office you are allowed to earn up to £35.00 doing work of therapeutic value without losing any benefit.

How to claim
After you have been ill for four days (not counting Sunday), apply on form SC.1 (which you get from a doctor's surgery or clinic) After this you will need to send a 'Doctor's Statement' every so often.

The statement will include the 'medical reason' for your not being able to work, but, at the most, this need relate only to the symptoms or opportunistic infection – 'pneumonia', for example. Doctors have to act in the best interests of their patients. If giving certain information is likely to cause stress or concern for the patient, the doctor is perfectly entitled to put down something much more neutral. The key is to talk to the doctor beforehand to see what is possible. If the DSS want a second opinion they may ask you to see a doctor from the Regional Medical Service; rules of confidentiality apply to this doctor as well.

More information
Leaflet NI.16 'Sickness Benefit'

YOU ARE NOT ABLE TO WORK BECAUSE YOU ARE ILL – AFTER 28 WEEKS (see general booklet FB.28 'Sick or disabled?')

IF YOU WERE PREVIOUSLY EMPLOYED OR SELF-EMPLOYED OR WERE UNEMPLOYED AND HAVE PAID SUFFICIENT NI CONTRI-BUTIONS

Invalidity Benefit (IVB)

Details
£46.90 tax-free, plus Earnings Related Pension, taxable. If this pension is less than £10.00, and you are under 40 when you become ill, the difference is paid as Invalidity Allowance and is tax-free.

Additions for dependants?
£9.65 for each child, tax-free, plus £28.20, tax-free, for an adult dependant who is earning less than £37.35.

Affected by periods in hospital?
Reduced by £18.80 after six weeks in hospital, or by £9.40 if you have a dependant.

Passport to other benefits?
If you get Housing Benefit (HB) or Income Support (IS) – you will qualify for a Disability Premium of £15.40 (if you are single) or £22.10 (if you are one of a couple) – see page 166 for HB and page 163 for IS.

Other notes
With the agreement of a doctor and the local Social Security office you are allowed to earn up to £35.00 doing work of therapeutic value without losing any benefit. £10 Christmas Bonus.

How to claim
After 22 weeks on Statutory Sick Pay your employer should give you a claim form to send to your local Social Security office. After 28 weeks of receiving Statutory Sick Pay or Sickness Benefit, payment of IVB should be automatic. If you have children, you may need to tell the Social Security office to make sure you get the extra for them. A doctor's statement is needed at regular intervals, unless your doctor sends a form to the DSS Regional Medical Officer to say that this is not necessary. The statement need not mention AIDS.

More information
Leaflet NI.16A 'Invalidity Benefit'

IF YOU HAVE NOT PAID SUFFICIENT NI CONTRIBUTIONS

Severe Disablement Allowance (SDA)

Details
£28.20, tax free. Can be payable if you have been incapable of work for at least 28 weeks. You must be 16 or over to qualify. If you became incapable of work *on or before your 20th birthday*, you do not have to have your disability assessed to get SDA. Up to total of 26 weeks work can be discounted. If you became incapable of work after your 20th birthday, you must also be assessed as at least 80% disabled. You will be treated as 80% disabled if:

- you are getting Attendance Allowance
- you are getting Mobility Allowance

- you are getting war pensioner's mobility supplement
- you have received a vaccine damage payment
- you have an invalid tricycle or invalid car or private car allowance from the Social Security
- you are registered as blind or partially sighted with a local authority in England or Wales or with a regional or islands council in Scotland
- you have already been found to be 80% disabled for Industrial Injuries Disablement Benefit or for War Disablement Pension.

If none of these descriptions applies to you, the DSS will ask a doctor to decide if you are 80% disabled. If you go back to work, or start work but fall ill again after a period of less than 8 weeks, you can reclaim SDA at once. If you fall ill after 8 weeks of working you have to wait for another 28 weeks to get SDA again.

Additions for dependants?
£9.65 for each child, tax-free, plus £16.65, taxable, for an adult dependant who is earning less than £37.35.

Affected by periods in hospital?
After six weeks in hospital, reduced by £18.80 or by £9.40 if you have a dependant.

Passport to other benefits?
If you can get Housing Benefit or Income Support – you will qualify for Disability Premium – see pages 151 and 166. £10 Christmas Bonus.

Other notes
You can't get Severe Disablement Allowance as well as Invalidity Benefit.

How to claim
Claim on form in leaflet NI.252.

In some cases, people who claim Severe Disablement Allowance will have the extent of their disability assessed by an adjudicating medical practitioner. This doctor is not concerned with the cause of the disability, and need not be told about the nature of the illness. There is no reason why the DSS should contact anyone about their decision or reasons for it.

More information
Leaflet NI.252 'Severe Disablement Allowance'

YOU ARE UNLIKELY EVER TO BE ABLE TO RETURN TO WORK

Incapacity Pension (IP)

The Civil Service, most public services and nationalised industries, as well as a few private companies, offer an Incapacity Pension to cover you when your Occupational Sick Pay comes to an end. This is in addition to any state contributory benefits. Means-tested benefits are affected.

Details
The amount (which is taxable) will depend on how long you have worked for the organisation and ranges from 12.5 per cent of your salary after five years service to 46 per cent after 30 years. You also get a tax-free lump sum equal to three times your initial annual pension.

Other notes
Some companies have a group Permanent Health Insurance or Salary Continuation Scheme instead. These pay at least half of your salary, no matter how long you have worked for the organisation.

How to claim and more information
Ask your employer or trade union.

YOU HAVE DIFFICULTY GETTING ABOUT (see general booklet HB.4 'Getting Around')

IF YOU ARE UNABLE OR ALMOST UNABLE TO WALK

Mobility Allowance (MA)

Details
£26.25 a week, tax-free, awarded to severely disabled people aged 5 to 65 if their mobility difficulty is likely to continue for at least 12 months (whatever the life expectancy). Claims must be received before age 66. MA can be paid to age of 80. It depends on a medical examination by a DSS doctor – see how to claim below. You can spend the allowance on what you like – not necessarily on transport.

Affected by periods in hospital?
No, unless you can't be moved for medical reasons, in which case it stops.

Passport to other benefits?
If you can get Housing Benefit or Income Support, you will qualify for a Disability Premium – see pages 151 and 166. The MA Unit should automatically send you an application for a certificate which exempts you from Vehicle Excise Duty (Road Tax). If they don't, ask for one. MA also qualifies you for parking concessions under the Orange Badge Scheme and a Disabled Person's Railcard (see below).

Other notes
MA is paid in full on top of all other benefits, and is not treated as income when calculating any HB, IS or Family Credit (FC) you may be entitled to. You can get MA whether or not you are working.

How to claim
Apply on form in leaflet NI.211 to MA Unit, DSS, Blackpool. Appeal if your first application is unsuccessful.

The DSS will arrange for a local doctor to see you at the surgery or at home. The doctor's report, is based only on your ability to walk and takes no account of the cause. You may, however, find the examination a gruelling experience. After this an adjudication officer makes a decision based on the doctor's report.

More information
Leaflet NI.211 'Mobility Allowance'

OTHER HELP WITH TRANSPORT

There are a number of other schemes to help with the cost of transport. The *Orange Badge Parking Scheme* allows you to park free at parking meters, and for up to two hours in most areas where parking is otherwise restricted – apply to your local Social Services department. Leaflet from library, CAB or Social Services. Most local authorities have some *concessionary fare scheme* for local public transport – again apply to Social Services. If you receive Mobility Allowance you will be eligible for a *Disabled Persons Railcard*. This will cost you £12, but will entitle you and a companion to worthwhile discounts on rail fares. If you live in Greater London, can't use public transport, and are able to use a 'black cab' you can join the *London Taxicard Scheme* which means you will be charged £1 for any taxi journey costing up to £7.60; for journeys which cost more than £7.60 you pay the extra (it does not apply in Redbridge and Barnet who have their own scheme). Leaflet and application form from any Post Office. And finally, if a continuing disability prevents you leaving home without help, you will be able to get *free prescriptions*. Apply on form in Leaflet P.11 'NHS Prescriptions'.

YOU ARE BLIND OR PARTIALLY SIGHTED see large print booklet FB.19 'A guide for blind and partially sighted people'

If a hospital eye specialist says that you are blind or partially sighted, you can ask your local Social Services Department to register you as such. Being registered helps get you the following benefits:

- loss of sight counts as sickness for Sickness and Invalidity Benefits if you need sight for your job
- Severe Disablement Allowance (see page 151)
- Disability Premium or Disabled Child Premium if on Income Support or Housing Benefit (see page 151)
- Orange Badge Parking Scheme (see page 154)
- Income Support from age 16 (see page 165)
- Disabled Persons Railcard (see page 154)
- Concessions on local transport (see page 137)
- Blind Persons Income Tax Allowance of £540, worth £2.60 a week to standard rate tax payers (see Inland Revenue leaflet IR.22)

YOU NEED SOMEONE AROUND TO HELP

Attendance Allowance (AA)

Details
If you need a lot of looking after by another person because you are mentally or physically disabled, you may be able to get AA. It is a weekly, tax-free benefit paid to you yourself and not to the person looking after you. You can get AA even if there is nobody to look after you. AA is paid at the rate of £25.05 if you need looking after day *or* night and at £37.55, if you need looking after day *and* night.

Affected by periods in hospital?
Benefit stops after you have been in hospital for four weeks

Passport to other benefits?
If you can get Housing Benefit or Income Support – you will qualify for a Disability Premium – see pages 151 and 166. If you are getting Attendance Allowance, a person who is caring for you may be able to get Invalid Care Allowance – see page 157.

Other notes
Attendance Allowance is generally paid in full on top of all other benefits, and is not treated as income when calculating any HB, IS or FC you may be entitled to (but see page 164). You can get AA whether you are working or not. However if you are resident in a private nursing or residential care home and in receipt of IS, AA will be taken into account in full when assessing your entitlement to IS. You can get AA whether you are working or not. You will also be entitled to a £10 Christmas bonus, unless you already get it with another benefit.

How to claim
Claim on form DS2 which is included in Leaflet NI.205. Send to appropriate regional office listed on the back of leaflet. Appeal if your first application is unsuccessful. The DSS will arrange for a doctor to see the applicant in his or her own home, but the report is based only on your needs, and takes no account of the cause of them. You may, however, find this examination a gruelling experience. A decision will be made by another doctor on the basis of the report and any other evidence you send in.

More information
Leaflet NI.205 'Attendance Allowance'

IF YOU ARE SEVERELY DISABLED AND HAVING TO *PAY* FOR SPECIAL CARE OR SPECIAL EQUIPMENT

Details
If you are getting Attendance Allowance, and you need extra cash for care or equipment which make it possible for you to live in the community rather than in special accommodation, you can apply for regular or one-off payments from the Government-funded Independent Living Fund. Write to ILF, PO Box 183, Nottingham, NG8 3RD (Tel. 0602 290423) for form ILF 100 if you are aged 16 or over; otherwise for form ILF 200. Payments from this fund are tax-free and are not counted as either income or capital for assessment of means-tested benefits.

IF YOU ARE LIVING ALONE AND GET ATTENDANCE ALLOWANCE (and no one gets Invalid Care Allowance to look after you).

When you are claiming Housing Benefit or Income Support (see pages 165–6) you can get a Severe Disability Premium of £28.20 in addition to the ordinary Disability Premium. You can still get this even if you have a carer living with you arranged by a voluntary organisation, to which you pay your Attendance Allowance.

IF YOU ARE LOOKING AFTER SOMEONE

Invalid Care Allowance (ICA)

Details
£28.20, taxable, for anyone under pension age who does not earn more than £20 after deductions of related expenses and spends at least 35 hours a week looking after someone who is getting Attendance Allowance. ICA can't be paid if you are receiving the same or a higher amount from certain other benefits. However it may still be worth claiming because you could qualify for the new carer's premium of £10 – see page 165.

Additions for dependants?
£9.65 for each child, tax-free, plus £16.65, for an adult dependant, taxable, who is earning less than £16.85.

Other notes
If you give up work to look after someone who is getting Attendance Allowance, you can apply for Income Support to top up your ICA – see page 165. ICA will be taken into account in assessing entitlement to IS. While you are getting ICA you will be credited with NI contributions unless you are a married woman with a reduced contribution record. You will get the £10 Christmas bonus.

How to claim
Claim on form DS700 in Leaflet NI.212 to ICA unit DSS, Palatine House, Lancaster Road, Preston, Lancs PR1 1NS

More information
Leaflet NI.212 'Invalid Care Allowance'

WHEN SOMEONE DIES (see booklet FB29 'Help When Someone Dies')

FUNERAL EXPENSES

Details
Anyone getting Income Support, Family Credit, Housing Benefit or Community Charge Rebate who has to arrange a funeral, can get money from the Social Fund to cover essential items. Any savings you have in excess of £500 (£1000 if aged 60 or over) will be deducted from this amount. Note that this has to be repaid from the estate of the dead person if there is enough money to do so. The value of a house left to a spouse does not count in calculating the value of an estate for this purpose.

How to claim
On form SF.200 from your local Social Security office.

IF YOU ARE WIDOWED

Income Tax Allowance

Details
In addition to the normal personal allowances, there is a Widow's Bereavement Allowance of £1590 (worth an extra £7.64 a week for standard rate tax payers) for the tax year of the husband's death and for the year after. If there is a dependent child, either widow or widower also gets an Additional Allowance of £1590.

How to claim
By letter to your tax office.

More information
Inland Revenue leaflet IR.23

Social Security benefits
Leaflet NP.45 'A Guide to Widows' Benefits'

Widow's Payment

Details
£1,000 tax-free lump sum to all those widowed aged under 60, and those aged 60 if their late husband was not receiving Retirement Pension, depending on the husband's NI contribution record.

How to claim
To your local Social Security office, using the form on the back of a special Social Security death certificate which the Registrar will give you, or in a letter saying you wish to claim Widow's Payment.

Widowed Mother's Allowance

Details
£46.90 taxable plus £9.65 tax free for each dependent child for those widowed with dependent children, depending on your late husband's NI contribution record

How to apply
As for Widow's Payment above.

Widow's Pension

Details
For those widowed at age 45 or over when widowed or when Widowed Mother's Allowance ends, and without dependent children. £46.90 taxable if aged 55 or over, less if you are widowed younger, down to zero if age less than 45.

How to claim
As for Widow's Payment above.

Widow's Additional Pension

Details
If your late husband had been paying into the state earnings related pension scheme, you will get an additional pension based on his earnings since 1978. If he was 'contracted out' of the state scheme, you will get about half the amount.

How to claim
No need; you will get it automatically when you claim your other widow's benefits.

Occupational Pension

Details
Most pension schemes pay a pension to a widow, some also to widowers. Amounts vary from scheme to scheme.

How to claim & more information
Ask your spouse's employer.

MATERNITY AND CHILDREN

HAVING A BABY – See booklets FB8 'Babies and Benefits' and FB27 'Bringing Up Children'

Statutory Maternity Pay (SMP)

Paid for 18 weeks after you stop work. To get this you must stop work at any time between 11 and six weeks before your baby is due.

Details
If you have worked full-time for your employer for two years up to 15 weeks before your baby is due: 90 per cent of your earnings for the first 6 weeks, then £39.25 for 12 weeks, both subject to tax and NI contributions. If you have worked for the same employer for between six months and 2 years, you get £39.25 for all the 18 weeks.

How to claim
From your employer at least three weeks before you stop work. Give him your maternity certificate MAT.B1 which you can get from a doctor or midwife.

More information
Leaflet NI.17A 'Maternity Benefits'

Maternity Allowance

If you don't qualify for SMP (see above), but have paid enough NI contributions.

Details
£35.70, tax-free for 18 weeks after you stop work, which must be between 11 and six weeks before your baby is due.

How to claim
On form MA.1 from your clinic to your local Social Security office.

More information
Leaflet NI.17A 'Maternity Benefits'

Free Prescriptions and dental treatment

Given while you are pregnant and for 12 months after the birth.

How to claim
On form FW.8 from your clinic or doctor.

More information
Leaflets P.11 'NHS Prescriptions' and D.11 'NHS Dental Treatment'

Maternity Payment

Details
If you are getting Income Support or Family Credit – £100 lump sum, tax-free, less the amount of any savings you have over £500.

How to claim
Paid from the Social Fund. Claim on form SF.100 from your clinic to your local Social Security office.

Child Benefit

Details
£7.25, tax-free for each child under 16, under 19 if in full-time relevant education.

How to claim
For a new baby you can get the right claim form by using the coupon in booklet FB.8, otherwise ask your local Social Security office for a claim form – they will need to know if you are getting Child Benefit for another child.

More information
Leaflet CH.1 'Child benefit'

One Parent Benefit

Details
£5.60, tax-free for the eldest child on top of Child Benefit.

Other notes
If you are a widowed mother, claim Widowed Mother's Allowance instead.

How to claim
Leaflets FB.8 or CH.11 or by letter to your local Social Security office.

More information
Leaflet CH.11 'One parent benefit'

Additional Tax Allowance

Details
An unmarried parent who is looking after a child, even if living with a partner, can get an extra allowance of £1590, worth £7.64 a week if you pay standard rate income tax.

How to claim
Apply to your tax office.

More information
Inland Revenue leaflet IR.22

IF YOUR CHILD IS SERIOUSLY ILL OR DISABLED

Details
Some benefits are available for children and young people in their own right:

Attendance Allowance.
Mobility Allowance from age five.
Severe Disablement Allowance from age 16.
Income Support from age 16, if incapable of work, registered blind or is a lone parent (otherwise from age 18).
Free pint of milk a day, if not registered at a school.

Families with a disabled child get an extra Premium of £15.40 when calculating entitlement to Income Support or Housing Benefit.

The *Family Fund* is a Government Fund administered by the Joseph Rowntree Memorial Trust, to help families with a very severely handicapped child under 16 years of age. Help given includes equipment, family holidays, outings, driving lessons, clothing, bedding, recreational and other items. Apply giving the child's full name, age, address, details of handicap, and help needed to: The Family Fund, PO Box 50, York, YO1 1UY.

IF YOU HAVE HAEMOPHILIA

Details
Single and weekly payments to meet special needs of those who develop HIV diseases as a result of blood products therapy are available from the Government-funded *MacFarlane Trust*. The amount will vary according to circumstances. Payments will not affect a claim for Income Support or Housing Benefit. In addition, an ex-gratia one-time payment of £20,000 will be made irrespective of means.

How to claim and more information
Apply to the MacFarlane Trust at PO Box 627, London SW1 0QG. Tel. 01-233 0342 (between 2pm–5pm)

INFECTED AT WORK

Details
In the extremely unlikely event that you become infected during the course of your work, you may have a case for getting Industrial Injuries Disablement Benefit if you develop AIDS. This benefit pays up to £76.60 in addition to Sickness or Invalidity Benefit.

More information
Leaflet NI.6 'Industrial Injuries Disablement Benefit'

INJURED BY CRIME

Should you suffer injury as a result of a crime of violence, you may be able to get compensation for pain and suffering, loss of earnings and some out of pocket expenses from the government-funded Criminal Injuries Compensation Board. To get compensation, it has to be assessed at £550 or more and you have to report the incident to the police without delay. The Board will obtain medical information from the doctor who treated you for your injuries. Any social security payments or other compensation you get because of the injury will be deducted.

How to apply
To the Criminal Injuries Compensation Board, Whittington House, 19 Alfred Place, London, WC1E 7LG. Tel 01-636 2812/9501.

Further information
Ask at your library or CAB for the Board's leaflet, 'Victims of crimes of violence'.

IF YOU GO INTO RESIDENTIAL CARE, A NURSING HOME OR HOSPICE

Details
If your savings are less than £6000, Income Support (see page 165) will top up

your income to £210 (£233 in Greater London) a week for residential care or up to £245 (£278 in Greater London) a week for a nursing home plus a Personal Allowance of £10.55. The home must be registered with the local council.

Other notes
These payments are means tested as part of Income Support, except that Attendance Allowance is regarded as income for this purpose.

How to claim
In writing to your local Social Security office and Social Services Department.

Community Charge (Poll Tax) Rebates and Exemptions

With the introduction of individual responsibility to pay, there is an individual entitlement for those on a low income to a rebate of up to 80%, depending on circumstances. All full-time students are entitled to the maximum rebate. Apply to your local Council, or via your local DSS office if you are getting Income Support. In addition, irrespective of income, you are totally exempt if your are a long-stay hospital patient or if you are being looked after in a nursing home, residential care home or in a hostel providing high levels of care. You should tell your local Council each time you go into and out of such care. A volunteer care worker looking after you, who gets low pay from a charity, is also exempt.

IF YOU HAVE A LOW INCOME

All the following benefits are for people on a low income. They are all means tested. This means that the *maximum* amount the law says you need depends on your particular circumstances – whether you are single or living with a partner, the ages of your children and what your housing costs are, for example. It also means that the amount of benefit you *actually get* is worked out by subtracting the income you and your partner are already getting from the maximum amount of benefit you are entitled to.

The exact rules are complicated and vary between the three different benefits – Income Support, Housing Benefit and Family Credit. So the application forms are lengthy and ask detailed questions about yourself, your household, your other circumstances, your savings and income from all other sources. For Income Support and Housing Benefit you also have to tell the authorities each time your circumstances change. For Family Credit you have to submit new details every six months.

INCOME SUPPORT

Details
If you are 18 or over (16 or over if unfit for work) you can claim if neither you nor your partner★ is working for 24 hours or more a week and your joint savings are less than £6000. Income Support brings your income up to what the law says people in different circumstances need to live on. It can be paid on top of any other benefit if need be.

If you are getting Unemployment Benefit your Income Support will be taxed; otherwise it is tax-free. The non-means tested benefits listed on pages 145–6, except Attendance and Mobility Allowance, count as income when the amount of Income Support you will get is being calculated. Any savings over £3000 are assumed to give you an income of £1 a week for each £250 (or part of).

Affected by periods in hospital?
Reduces *to* £11.75 after six weeks in hospital if you are single or *by* £9.40 if you have a partner.

Other notes
If you get Income Support, you can also get the maximum Housing Benefit from your local council – see page 166. If you can't get Income Support, and your savings are less than £8000, you may still be able to get some Housing Benefit, although it won't be as much. The maximum amount of income support will rise by £10 from October 1990 for carers who get ICA, or who would get it if they didn't already have another higher benefit.

Passport to other benefits?
Getting Income Support gives you a 'passport' to the following benefits – free prescriptions, dental treatment, eye tests and vouchers for glasses, milk and vitamins for expectant mothers and children under five, refund of fares to hospital for treatment. You can also get Maternity Payment (£100 less the amount of any savings over £500) and the costs of a simple funeral (less the amount of any

★   Husband or wife, or someone of the opposite sex with whom you live as husband and wife. Benefit law explicitly excludes a homosexual relationship as a partnership.

savings over £500 or £1000 if aged 60 or over) from the Social Fund (see below). Children are eligible for free school meals and you may be eligible for Community Care Grants and Budgeting Loans from the Social Fund. You also qualify for a loft insulation grant. If your savings are less than £890 you can get free legal advice and assistance.

How to claim
By letter or on form in leaflet SB.1 to your local Social Security office. But if you are unemployed, get form B1 from your Unemployment Benefit office.

More information
Leaflet SB.1 and Booklet SB.20

Disability Premium

If you or your partner are getting Invalidity Benefit, Severe Disablement Allowance, Mobility Allowance or Attendance Allowance or are registered blind, you will qualify for a Disability Premium of £15.40 if you are single or £22.10 if you are married or live with a partner.(£17.05 or £24.25 respectively if the disabled person is 60 or over.) To get this tell your Social Security office.

If you, or your partner have been off work due to sickness and have been sending in doctor's statements covering 28 weeks, you can get the Disability Premium even if you are not getting any of the benefits listed above.

HOUSING BENEFIT

Details
For anyone who pays rent or poll tax, and whose savings are less than £8000. If on Income Support, you get maximum Housing Benefit – 100 per cent of rent and 80 per cent of poll tax. Otherwise your needs are assessed in the same way as for Income Support. If you or your partner are getting Invalidity Benefit, Severe Disablement Allowance, Mobility Allowance or Attendance Allowance or are registered blind, you will qualify for an extra Disability Premium of £15.40 if you are single or £22.10 if you are married or live with a partner (£17.05 or £24.25 respectively if the disabled person is 60 or over).

Additions
Various extra allowances for children, partner, if you are disabled, blind, a lone parent, have a disabled child or are aged 60 or over.

Affected by periods in hospital?
Stops after a year in hospital, but can then be claimed by partner.

Passport to other benefits?
Loft insulation grant; funeral payment from Social Fund.

Other notes
You will get somewhat less if you have an adult non-dependant living in your household, or if your rent includes a charge for fuel. The maximum amount of Housing Benefit will rise by £10 from October 1990 for carers who get ICA or who would get it if they didn't already have another higher benefit.

How to claim
On form from DSS if you are getting Income Support; otherwise on a form from your local council.

More information
Leaflet RR.1 and Booklet RR.2

IF ANOTHER ADULT LIVES IN YOUR HOUSEHOLD, WHO IS NOT FINANCIALLY DEPENDENT ON YOU

Housing Benefit you get as a householder and any housing costs you get as part of Income Support are normally reduced if there is a 'non-dependent' adult (such as grown-up children or elderly relatives) living in the household. If you are blind or getting Attendance Allowance, tell your local Council and Social Security office and your benefits will not be reduced.

INCOME SUPPORT AND HOUSING BENEFIT WHILE LIVING AWAY FROM YOUR HOME

Board & Lodging and Hostels

You have to apply to the DSS for Income Support and to the local Council for Housing Benefit; the standard allowances, premiums and other rules apply (see above). You can get Housing Benefit Rent Allowance in advance if moving into new accommodation, but Income Support is paid in arrears, one week if you are incapable of work, two weeks if you have to sign on. If you have no cash available it is worthwhile applying for a crisis loan from the DSS Social Fund (see page 170) until you get your Housing Benefit and Income Support.

Residential Care Homes

Your benefit is paid by the DSS. The assessment is made up of an allowance for personal expenses of £10.55 and your accommodation charge varying from £150 to £210 (depending on the care you need) plus a maximum of £23 in the Greater London area.

The amount of benefit paid is the amount of your assessment less your other resources, and you cannot claim if your savings are more than £6000. The whole of any Attendance Allowance is regarded as part of your resources.

Partners and dependants living at home will receive the standard premium, mortgage interest, if applicable, and the maximum Housing Benefit. These arrangements apply for both long and short stays. If your savings are more than £6000, so that you can't get Income Support, spending some of your savings on your accommodation will not prevent you claiming IS as soon as they fall to £6000. If you previously lived alone in your own home, its value will not be counted as capital for Income Support for the first 26 weeks (or possibly longer) if you are trying to sell it.

Nursing Homes

Benefit arrangements are as for Residential Care Homes (see above) except that the maximum charge allowed is £245 if you are physically disabled or have a terminal illness (again plus £23 in Greater London).

Hospitals

Your full Income Support and Housing Benefit continues unaltered for periods of up to 6 weeks in hospital. Periods separated by 28 days or less at home count as a single period for the operation of the six week rule.

Reduces to £11.75 after six weeks in hospital if you are single or by £9.40 if you have a partner.

Any IS housing costs (such as mortgage interest) payments continue. If your IS is reduced to nothing, you will have to re-apply for Housing Benefit. If you have a partner at home, he or she can claim HB instead of you. Otherwise Housing Benefit will continue for 12 months and then stop.

FAMILY CREDIT

Details
Paid, tax-free, if you or your partner are working 24 hours or more a week, you have one or more dependent children under 16 or 16–19 in full-time education up to A-level or equivalent, and your savings are no more than £6000. Amount depends on your net income and on the number and age of your children. Family Credit is not a loan and does not have to be paid back. You will get a fixed amount for 26 weeks, after which you have to apply again.

Affected by periods in hospital?
Once made, an award of Family Credit continues for 26 weeks regardless of stays in hospital.

Passport to other benefits?
Getting Family Credit automatically gives you the following benefits: free prescriptions, free dental treatment, eye tests and vouchers for glasses, refund of fares to hospital for treatment. You can get a Maternity Payment (£100 less the amount of any savings over £500) and the cost of a simple funeral (less the amount of any savings over £500 or £1000 if aged 60 or over), from the Social Fund. If you have savings of less than £890 you can also get free legal advice and assistance. You also qualify for a loft insulation grant.

How to claim
On claim form in leaflet FC.1. available from post offices and local DSS offices

More information
Leaflet NI.261 'A guide to Family Credit'

FREE NHS CHARGES – General leaflet AB.11 'Help with NHS costs'

Details
Even if your family income is somewhat too high for you to qualify for Income Support or Family Credit and your savings are no more than £6000, you may still be able to get free prescriptions (currently £2.80 an item) and free or reduced charges for dental treatment, help with the cost of a sight test, vouchers for spectacles, NHS wigs and fabric supports and refunds of fares to and from hospital either as an out-patient or as an in-patient.

How to apply
To DSS Newcastle upon Tyne, on form AG1 available from dentists, opticians, hospitals or your local Social Security office. If you qualify you will receive a certificate of entitlement which lasts for six months and which gives details of the amount of help you may get. Remember, you can't get a refund for glasses unless prescribed by a hospital, and other refunds must be claimed within one month of paying a charge.

More information
Special leaflets telling you who gets these services free automatically and how to work out if your income is low enough to qualify.

P.11 'NHS Prescriptions' from GPs
D.11 'NHS Dental treatment' from dentists
G.11 'NHS Vouchers for glasses' from opticians
H.11 'NHS Hospital travel costs' from hospitals
WF.11 'NHS Wigs and fabric supports' from hospitals
or from your local Social Security office

MONEY FROM THE SOCIAL FUND

The Social Fund provides grants and interest-free loans. These are designed to help people getting Income Support to meet the cost of extra expenses which are difficult to pay for out of regular income (more information in Booklet SB.16). Each DSS office has its own budget and system of priorities and there is no independent right of appeal.

Funeral Payment
If you are getting Housing Benefit or Community Charge Rebate, Family Credit or Income Support you will be eligible for the cost of essential funeral expenses, less the cost of any savings you have over £500 (£1000 if aged 60 or over). The payment has to be paid back from the dead person's estate if there's enough money to do so. (A house left to a spouse is not included in the estate for this purpose).

How to claim
Form SF200 from your local Social Security office or the registrar.

More information
Booklet FB.29 'Help when someone dies'

Maternity Payment
Any parent getting Family Credit or Income Support can get £100, tax-free, less the amount of any savings you have over £500.

How to claim
Contact your local Social Security office for a claim form.

More information
Booklet FB.8 'Babies and benefits'

Cold Weather Payment
If you are getting Income Support for a child under five, or for someone who is disabled or over 60, or for a disabled child, you can get £5 for each very cold seven days (when the average temperature is 0°C/32°F or lower), less the amount of any savings you have over £500, £1000 if aged 60 or over.

How to claim
Contact your local Social Security office or look for announcements in the press.

More information
Leaflet SB.17A 'Extra help with heating costs'

Community Care Grant
If you get Income Support, you can apply for money which will make it possible for you to live at home rather than in residential care. Grants are discretionary; the amount given will depend on individual circumstances and are less any savings you have over £500, (£1000 if aged 60 or over). These do not have to be repaid.

How to claim
Contact your local Social Security office.

Budgeting loan
If you have been getting Income Support for 6 months, you can apply for an interest-free loan to help pay for specific items you need like furniture, household equipment and home repairs. Such loans are discretionary and depend on your

individual circumstances, and are less the amount of any savings you have over £500 (£1000 if aged 60 or over). The loan is repaid by making deductions from your benefit payments.

How to claim
Apply to your local Social Security office.

Crisis loan
Awarded for emergency situations when no offer of help is immediately available. You do not have to be getting Income Support.

How to claim
Apply to your local Social Security office.

Unhappy with your benefit

If you think a decision about your benefit is wrong, you can ask for a 'review'. You can do this if you think you have been refused a benefit you consider you are entitled to, or if you feel the amount is too low.

For Family Credit, Income Support, Funeral Payments and Maternity Payments you can also appeal to a Tribunal where you will be able to make your case personally. Appealing is often successful. To appeal, write a letter giving details of why you think the decision was wrong. Advice centres such as the Citizens Advice Bureau will help you with the details, and will sometimes go to a tribunal with you. This may improve your chances of success. See Leaflet NI.246 'How to appeal' and Booklet NI.260 'A guide to reviews and appeals'.

WHERE TO FIND MORE DETAILS OF INDIVIDUAL BENEFITS

Leaflets and Guides

All DSS benefits are described in leaflets which give details of who is eligible and how to claim. Most of the leaflets don't give the actual amount of each benefit, because these change every year. Details of these are published separately each March in leaflet NI.196 'Social Security benefit rates'.

All leaflets are available free from libraries, Citizens Advice Bureaux (CABx) and DSS offices; some are available from post offices or the address below:

DSS Leaflet Unit
PO Box 21
Stanmore
Middlesex, HA7 1AY

Because of the new system which started in April 1988, make sure you get hold of up to date editions. Most leaflets are only updated following a change to the rules, so it can be difficult to tell if you have the latest version – ask your Social Security office or call freephone 0800-666 555 (England, Scotland, Wales), 0800-616757 (Northern Ireland), for the date of the latest version if you are in any doubt. Subsequent editions of the same leaflet always have the same reference number as the earlier version.

Starting points

Booklet FB.2, called *Which benefit?*, gives a summary of each benefit and will help you identify those which might apply to you. Three other very useful general leaflets are:

NI.196   Social Security benefit rates – published in March each year, gives the amount of each benefit.

NI.9   Going into hospital? – explains how your benefits are affected if you go into hospital for a short stay or long term.

NI.246   How to appeal – what to do if you feel you should be getting a benefit which the DSS tells you you are not eligible for.

Benefits for different groups of people

A series of booklets give brief details of benefits for different groups of people or for different situations:

HB. 1   Help for handicapped people
HB. 2   Equipment for disabled people
HB. 4   Getting around, help with mobility
FB. 4   Cash help while you are working
FB. 6   Retiring?
FB. 8   Babies and benefits
FB. 9   Unemployed?

FB.23   Young people's guide to social security
FB.27   Bringing up children?
FB.28   Sick or disabled?
FB.29   Help when someone dies
FB.30   Self-employed?

For details of the new benefits introduced in April 1988, and how they are worked out, there is a series of Fact Sheets:

FIG.2   Income Support
FIG.3   Family Credit
FIG.4   The Social Fund
FIG.5   Housing Benefit
FIG.6   Widow's Benefits

See also fact sheet FC.2 for Family Credit in leaflet FC.1

For detailed leaflets, see those listed under 'more information for each individual benefit'.

More comprehensive details are given in a series of larger Guide Books:

SB.20   A Guide to Income Support
RR.2   A Guide to Housing Benefits
NI.261   A Guide to Family Credit
SB.16   A Guide to the Social Fund
NI.17A   A Guide to Maternity Benefits
NP.45   A Guide to Widows' Benefits
HB.5   A Guide to non-Contributory benefits for disabled people
FB.19   A Guide for blind and partially sighted people.
NI.260   A Guide to Reviews and Appeals

For really comprehensive and exhaustive information, look at: 'Disability Rights Handbook' published annually in May by the Disability Alliance ERA, 25 Denmark Street, London WC2H 8NJ, (price £3.75 post free). Updated information is given three times a year in the Disability Rights Bulletin.

'National Welfare Benefits Handbook', by the Child Poverty Action Group, 1–5 Bath Street, London EC1V 9PY, (price £5.50 post free, 1989/90 issue; cheques/POs payable to CPAG Ltd) and 'Rights Guide to Non-Means Tested Benefits', also by the Child Poverty Action Group, at the same address, (price £4.95 post free, 1989/90 issue; cheques/POs payable to CPAG Ltd). Updated information for both books is given six times a year in the Bulletin. Your public library should have these.

Collecting benefits

If you are unable to get to a post office to cash an order in your benefit book, someone else can cash it for you. You have to fill in his or her name on the back of each order and sign where indicated.

If you are drawing benefit and are unable to get to a post office for some time, you can nominate someone as your 'agent' to collect your benefits regularly. Ask your Social Security office to issue him or her with a card to show the post office each time.

If you are likely to be in and out of hospital and need to claim benefit each time you are at home, you can tell your Social Security office you want to nominate someone as your 'appointee'. This enables the appointee to act for you in telling the DSS each time you go into and come out of hospital and to claim benefits on your behalf. In effect the appointee becomes the claimant and he or she must inform the DSS of any change of circumstances. Ask your Social Security office for form BF.56.

Special funds and charities

The following organisations give grants (and sometimes equipment) to people with ARC or AIDS. Unless we say otherwise they will also consider the needs of people who are HIV-positive. Applications can usually be made by people with AIDS, carers, or professionals such as GPs or social workers. Where special information is needed we give details.

You should also check your local AIDS helpline (see page 295). Some may make grants directly or know of local or new sources not listed here. You may also want to approach charities which give funds to people in need generally, rather than those set up solely to help with HIV. These are listed in the following publications – your local library might have copies; if not they should be able to tell you which other local library does.

> *Charities Digest*
> Publisher: The Family Welfare Association
> Lists charitable trusts and associations
>
> *Directory of Grant-Making Trusts*
> Publisher: Charities Aid Foundation
> Lists trusts in the UK
>
> *Directory of Grant-Making Trusts and Organisations in Scotland*
> Publisher: Scottish Council for Voluntary Organisations
> Lists local and national trusts and organisations in Scotland
>
> *Guide to Grants for Individuals in Need*
> Publisher: Directory of Social Change
> Lists about 1000 local charities which make grants to individuals, as well as national and general charities.

ACET

ACET is a charity which provides health education in schools, and training for professionals and the public. They also lend equipment and make grants to cover the cost of an item or bill that cannot easily or quickly be met by the Social Fund (see page 170 for details of the Social Fund). These include furniture, electrical equipment, the installation of a telephone and – occasionally – money towards holidays. Most grants so far awarded have been between £100 and £200. ACET have just started a lending 'library' of microwave ovens and fridges; they hope to extend this to other electrical equipment.

ACET (AIDS, care, education and training)

PO Box 1323
London W5 5TF
01-840 7879

PO Box 147
Portsmouth PO2 9DA
(0705) 693422

PO Box 153
Dundee DD1 9RH
(0382) 202463

PO Box 108
Edinburgh EH8 9NY
031-6684225

AIDS AHEAD

AIDS AHEAD is a charity which provides health education and advice about AIDS for deaf people. It does not normally make grants but in cases of urgent need may lend a communicating terminal and might consider paying for a telephone to be installed.

AIDS AHEAD, c/o Cheshire Society for the Deaf
144 London Road
Northwich
Cheshire CW9 5HH   (0606) 47047

Aled Richards Trust

The Aled Richards Trust aims to help people directly affected by HIV, or, people in close relationships with them, who are living in and around Bath, Bristol and Weston-super-Mare. Grants are given for bills, furniture and alternative therapies. PWAs should apply themselves and need to be able to give confirmation of the diagnosis from a GP, social worker or other professional. The average grant is £100 and there is an upper limit of £500 for each person in any one year.

Aled Richards Trust
54 Colston Street
Bristol BS1 5AZ   (0272) 297963
Helpline (0272) 273436 (Monday to Friday, 7pm to 9pm)

Body Positive

Body Positive makes small grants to people who are HIV-positive. They will consider applications for such things as furniture, kitchen equipment, bedding, clothing, travel expenses, telephone installation, fuel bills and alternative health care. Applications should be accompanied by a letter from a doctor or social worker who can confirm the diagnosis. The maximum awarded is usually £200. Most grants are one-off although, under special circumstances, the panel will consider exceeding the £200 limit or giving additional grants. Other Body Positive groups may also be able to help.

Body Positive Small Grants Fund
PO Box 493
London W14 0TF   01-835 1045

CHART

CHART is a self-funding organisation which makes grants to people who are HIV-positive, or who have ARC or AIDS. Applications must be made through a buddy (see page 68), social worker or doctor. Grants are given to pay for tangible items such as heating bills and kitchen equipment. They are not likely to be more than £100.

CHART (Customers helping AIDS relief trust)
PO Box 2236
London W14 9EW   01-381 1731

CRUSAID

CRUSAID have an Individual Hardship Fund to help people who are HIV-positive, or have ARC or AIDS and who are in financial difficulties as a result of their illness. The fund pays for such things as telephone installations, furnishings (where someone has been rehoused), and essential equipment such as washing machines. Applications should be made by a doctor, social worker, health advisor or buddy to CRUSAID by phone or in writing. The average grant is £125. Each case will be assessed on the degree of need and financial hardship.

CRUSAID
83 Clerkenwell Road
London EC1R 5AR   01-831 2595

David Manley Fund

Leicestershire AIDS Support Services administers the David Manley Fund which gives direct financial help to people living in Leicestershire. Grants are given for a variety of reasons, including contributions towards such things as bills, fares to and from hospital, furniture, kitchen equipment and baby sitting. Applications should be made direct to LASS.

David Manley Fund
c/o Leicestershire AIDS Support Services
Leicester Council for Voluntary Services
32 De Montfort Street
Leicester LE1 7GD   (0533) 549922 (x6429)

Frontliners

Frontliners usually makes grants to people with AIDS themselves, but in some cases will pay for a carer to travel to visit or care for a person with AIDS. The grants can be used to pay bills, fund telephone installation, buy furniture or other essential household items etc. Referral from a professional or voluntary body is not necessary although would be accepted. Self-referral is encouraged. A letter of diagnosis is required before any grants are paid. The sums granted vary according to need.

Frontliners
52–54 Gray's Inn Road
London WC1X 8JU   01-831 0330

LEAN

London East AIDS Network give grants to people who live in the East London or inner Essex areas. They are usually one-off grants, up to a maximum of £150, for such things as furniture or installation of a telephone. Whenever possible cheques will be made out to the company supplying the goods rather than to a person with AIDS or carer. Applications must be made through a social worker or health visitor who can confirm the diagnosis. LEAN can also make emergency cash grants or loans; these would also have to be made through a third party. Grants to cover the travel costs of families visiting people in hospital may also be available.

London East AIDS Network
PO Box 243
London E6 3HL   01-519 7457

MacFarlane Trust

Single and weekly payments to meet special needs of people with haemophilia who develop an HIV illness as a result of blood products therapy are available from the Government-funded MacFarlane Trust. The amount will vary according to circumstances. In addition, an ex-gratia one-time payment of £20,000 will be made irrespective of means.

MacFarlane Trust
PO Box 627
London SW1 0QG   01-233 0342 (between 2pm and 5pm)

Macmillan Fund

The Cancer Relief Macmillan Fund Grants Department gives grants to help people with cancer who are in financial difficulties for practical things – heating, laundry and so on. Application must be made through a local authority or medical social worker, or community nursing staff.

The Macmillan Fund
Anchor House
15–19 Britten Street
London SW3 3TZ   01-351 7811

Mainliners

Mainliners will soon be relaunching their grants scheme for people with HIV. Money can be used to pay bills and buy necessary equipment and furniture. Applications by post only should be made by the person with AIDS; written confirmation of the diagnosis will be needed. Also required is information about what the grant is for, details of the person with AIDS' financial position, including any benefits being received. Grants will not be paid in cash. For people outside London the grant will be paid through a local organisation.

Mainliners
PO Box 125
London SW9 8EF   01-274 4000 (x354)

Malcolm Sargent Cancer Fund

The Malcolm Sargent Cancer Fund gives grants to young people under the age of 21 who have cancer, leukaemia, or Hodgkin's disease. You will need to fill in an application form and the diagnosis will have to be confirmed by a social worker, GP or other professional. Grants are given to help with the costs of travel, heating, holidays and clothing.

The Malcolm Sargent Cancer Fund for Children
14 Abingdon Road
London W8 6AF   01-837 4548

Marie Curie Cancer Care

People with cancer may be eligible for assistance from the Marie Curie Cancer Care's Welfare Grants Scheme. The grants are intended to give emergency help for items not available from the statutory services or other charities or where you would have to wait too long for help. Up to £50 can be awarded for such things as heaters, extra clothing, bed linen, fans and liquidisers. For further information contact your District Nurse or Community Nursing Officer.

Community Nursing Department
Marie Curie Cancer Care
28 Belgrave Square
London SW1X 8QG   01-235 3325

Monument Trust

The Monument Trust makes grants to people with HIV related illnesses and, occasionally, to carers. Grants are not usually for more than £250. Applications should be made in writing through a registered charity.

The Monument Trust
13 New Row
St Martin's Lane
London WC2N 4LF   01-836 6477/836 4619

OXAIDS

OXAIDS has a limited fund to make grants to people living in the Oxfordshire area. The grants can be used to pay for a variety of items. Applications should be made in writing and a letter confirming diagnosis will be needed. Each case is assessed on its merit and sums vary depending on need.

OXAIDS
c/o Radcliffe Infirmary
Woodstock Road
Oxford OX2 6HE   (0865) 728817

Positively Women Childrens' Fund

Positively Women give grants of up to £100 for each child of an HIV-positive mother. You will need a letter confirming diagnosis. For details contact:

Positively Women
333 Gray's Inn Road
London WC1X 8PX   01-837 9705

Salvation Army

The Salvation Army has two funds that make grants to people who are HIV-positive, have AIDS or ARC. The AIDS Fund is financed by the profits made from the sale of their book 'AIDS CARE'. Grants will be made for very small items, such as timers which remind people when to take their medicines. The Hypothermia Fund makes grants to help people keep warm – money for heaters, fuel bills and warm clothing, for example.

The Secretary (Mark all correspondence confidential)
Services to the Community
Salvation Army
101 Queen Victoria Street
London EC4P 4EP   01-236 5222

SAM

Scottish AIDS Monitor has two funds which make financial awards to people who are HIV-positive, who have AIDS or ARC and live in Scotland. The Hardship fund will give money for a variety of everyday needs including large electricity bills and the installation of telephones. The McKellen Fund can help pay towards holidays for people with AIDS or ARC, including the travel costs of a companion. Referral can be made by people with AIDS, a doctor, buddy, carer or social worker. Diagnosis must, however, be confirmed by a doctor. Each application will be considered on its own merit taking into consideration the applicant's circumstances and needs.

Scottish AIDS Monitor
PO Box 48
Edinburgh EH1 3SA   031-557 3885

Terrence Higgins Trust

The Terrence Higgins Trust has two funds which make grants. The No 1 Fund aims to help people with AIDS and ARC to improve the quality of their life. The No 2 Fund is for ex-offenders and drug users who are HIV-positive. Grants from both funds can be used for fuel bills (up to a maximum of £50 per quarter), telephone bills (up to £75 a quarter), travel, clothes, furniture and electrical equipment – although when possible these items will be lent by THT. Payments may also be made for up to four weeks while you are waiting for DSS benefits to be arranged. Grants of up to £100 may be made towards paying for a holiday if recommended for medical reasons.

Whenever possible cheques will be made out to the company or organisation supplying goods and services rather than to the individual involved. Confirmation of diagnosis will be needed along with information about income and expenditure. Grants do not generally exceed £200, but in cases of special need THT will co-operate with other sources of funding to help as much as possible.

No 1/No 2 Fund
Terrence Higgins Trust
52-54 Gray's Inn Road
London WC1X 8JU   01-831 0330

10 Symptoms and medical treatment

Symptoms

Debilitating symptoms in people with AIDS are common. Some are due to complications which set in because the body has been weakened by HIV and others are due to the HIV infection itself. Below we give brief details of the main symptoms associated with AIDS and ARC, the chief causes of these symptoms and notes on some current treatments. However, new treatments and new theories appear frequently and the precise treatment given to someone may depend on the hospital or clinic. See page 194 for how to get more information.

It should be stressed that these symptoms are not in themselves necessarily a sign of ARC or AIDS – they could be due to other causes. Diagnosis should always be made by a qualified person.

Current treatment

Constitutional symptoms

Constitutional symptoms are general signs of ill health which are attributed to HIV in the absence of any other illness which could explain them. They include fever, weight loss and/or diarrhoea. They occur both in people with ARC or AIDS and may be extremely debilitating. Night sweats and bouts of severe fatigue are also frequent complaints. Symptoms may be reduced by use of the drug zidovudine (previously known as AZT and often known by its brand name as Retrovir – see below). Other experimental therapies are also being tried. Some people have a persistent intermittent fever, with no apparent specific cause other than HIV. However, fever is often a sign of other infections which may be treatable. Many people with AIDS experience various general physical aches and pains.

Respiratory symptoms

The most common respiratory symptoms are coughs and breathlessness. There are several causes but by far the most common is a pneumonia caused by pneumocystis carinii.

Pneumocystis carinii
pneumonia (PCP)

This is the most common major opportunistic infection. (An opportunistic infection is one that would not normally get a hold on a healthy immune system but which occurs because a weakened system is less able to fight it.) Symptoms often develop gradually over one or two weeks and usually include a dry, persistent cough, increasing breathlessness, discomfort when breathing in and fevers. One in four people who had PCP used to die from it, but the majority of people now recover because of better methods of treatment and earlier diagnosis. If pneumocystis carinii pneumonia is suspected, medical help should be sought.

Diagnosis involves a chest x-ray and examination of blood and sputum specimens. In some cases where diagnosis has not been confirmed, or where there is doubt, a bronchoscopy (inspection of the bronchial tubes with a narrow fibre optic tube) is necessary.

Treatment involves oxygen to relieve breathlessness (breathed in through a mask) and drugs. Co-trimoxazole (brand name Septrin or Bactrim) is used most often. This is injected slowly over two or three hours into a vein or continuously over 24 hours. It can also be taken orally. There are often side effects, particularly as high doses of the drug are necessary. These include nausea and vomiting, allergic rashes and damage to the bone marrow. All these side effects disappear once you stop taking the drug. Pentamidine can be used as an alternative to co-trimoxazole. This can also be injected but is now more often given in an inhalation. However, this may not give a sufficiently strong dose for severe cases. Side effects can include a lowering of the blood sugar, and it may affect the kidneys. Occasionally, people who are severely ill are given a combination of intravenous pentamidine, co-trimoxazole and oral corticosteroids (these are produced in the cortex of the adrenal glands; they fight inflammation and other conditions; synthetic ones also exist). Trimethoprim is an alternative drug for people allergic to co-trimoxazole. Treatment for PCP is given for up to three weeks.

Pneumocystis carinii pneumonia often recurs, and for this reason people are offered drugs to prevent it. These consist of daily doses of co-trimoxazole, weekly doses of Fansidar (an antimicrobial), or doses of pentamidine which have to be inhaled once every two weeks. PCP can be prevented by such treatments as aerosol pentamidine. It has become increasingly common to give treatment to anyone with AIDS or ARC as a preventive measure (prophylaxis).

Other causes

Tuberculosis of the lung may occur. This seems to affect people who are or have been injecting drug-users most frequently. 'Ordinary' TB can be treated successfully; medication usually lasts for six to nine months. Other types of infection such as MAI are less responsive to treatment. These 'atypical' TB infections tend to occur later and may not always have symptoms. Respiratory symptoms may also be caused by lung tumours such as Kaposi's sarcoma and lymphomas (see below).

Gastrointestinal symptoms
Mouth and throat

Pain, discomfort, difficulties swallowing and soreness in the mouth and throat are frequent complaints. *Oral candida (thrush)* is a common cause and is one of the first signs of damage to the immune system. It usually appears as a white furry coating on the tongue or throat or as a sore, red or inflamed throat. It can make eating and swallowing difficult. Antifungal treatment such as amphotericin lozenges or nystatin oral solution is normally successful. Severe infections respond to treatment with other antifungal medicines such as ketoconazole or fluconazole. These are also used to stop the symptoms reappearing. If thrush is associated with swallowing difficulties the gullet may also be affected. This is known as *oesophageal candida*; other symptoms are pains in the front of the chest and fevers.

Mouth ulcers are also a common complaint, and can occur singly or in patches at any one time. They also make eating and swallowing difficult and painful. Oral barrier pastes or local anaesthetic lozenges help to relieve symptoms. *Ulcerative gingivitus* can cause receding and painful gums which bleed easily when brushed. Treatment by a dentist together with a course of antibiotics will help.

Gut

By far the most common problem with the gut is *diarrhoea*. This can be associated with weight loss and anorexia and affects people with ARC as well as those with AIDS. Causes include opportunistic infections, tumours and the various other conditions associated with HIV. For treatment to be effective the cause needs to be known. Investigations may be carried out without admission to hospital, but this may depend on the severity of symptoms. Investigations include examination of the faeces and/or a sample of tissue taken from the rectum for signs of infection, inspection of the rectum or x-ray. Often the cause of the diarrhoea cannot be found and treatment is then just aimed at relieving symptoms. These may be severe enough to mean going into hospital, especially if the person has lost a lot of weight, has a fever, is dehydrated or is vomiting a great deal.

One specific cause is cryptosporidiosis – an infection of the gut. Symptoms vary from a chronic, intermittent diarrhoea to an acute, severe, high-volume, watery diarrhoea which can also be associated with abdominal pain, fever, nausea and vomiting. In some cases it is possible to lose six or seven litres of diarrhoea a day, which means that bodily fluids are being lost as well as fluids taken in during the day. This can cause wasting and profound weakness. Treatment of cryptosporidial diarrhoea is difficult.

Other causes of diarrhoea, which are more amenable to treatment, are giardiasis, salmonellosis, campylobacter enteritis. These also affect people who have not been infected by HIV, but are apt to be more severe for people with AIDS. In later stages of illness diarrhoea can be caused by cytomegalovirus and atypical mycobacterial infection, and is much more difficult to treat. Occasionally gastrointestinal symptoms are due to Kaposi's sarcoma or small bowel lymphoma. Whatever the cause of diarrhoea, it is accompanied with a decreased absorption of food. If weight loss follows and persists, special attention must be paid to diet to ensure an adequate intake of calories in the form of proteins, carbohydrates and vitamins. High-energy and nutritionally complete drinks and vitamin supplements will help.

Neurological symptoms

Headaches, loss of sight, fits and psychological problems can occur.

Cytomegalovirus retinitis (CMV)

This can be devastating if left untreated, as it ultimately leads to blindness. It affects about five to ten per cent of people with AIDS, usually in the later stages of illness. Symptoms include partial loss of sight and/or blurred vision.

Treatment is given by injecting the drug ganciclovir or phosphonoformate (brand name Foscarnet). Treatment has to be continued indefinitely as the condition often reappears, leading to progressive loss of sight. Treatment can be carried out at home by the person with AIDS if he or she has good enough vision; otherwise it can be carried out by a carer. The hospital will give training. If ganciclovir is used it may affect the bone marrow so it is necessary to have a full blood count regularly. The hospital will arrange this. Phosphonoformate may affect the kidneys so is often given as an infusion over a 24-hour period. Experiments in giving doses intermittently are being carried out. People who are taking AZT may have to take a reduced dose while being treated for CMV.

Cryptococcal meningitis

The fungus cryptococcus neoformans causes a life-threatening meningitis (inflammation affecting the membranes of the brain, spinal cord or both). Signs are very severe headaches, vomiting, fever and photophobia (in which bright lights will cause discomfort). Diagnosis is confirmed by the finding of cryptococcus in the cerebral spinal fluid. Treatment involves intravenous therapy via a central vein of either amphotericin B and flucytosine or a recently developed drug called fluconazole. It is too early to say whether fluconazole will be effective in the long term. After this, regular treatment with either intravenous amphotericin B or an oral preparation of fluconazole is needed to prevent a relapse.

Cerebral toxoplasmosis

Toxoplasma gondii – sometimes known colloquially as 'toxo' – is an organism that invades the nervous system, and can cause abscesses in the brain. Symptoms are severe headaches, high fevers, confusion and, later on, seizures, gradual weakness or paralysis of one side of the body and occasional loss of consciousness. This condition is serious and can cause rapid deterioration. A scan of the brain is needed to confirm the diagnosis; sometimes, it is necessary to examine tissue taken from the brain. Treatment is usually by a combination of sulphadiazine and pyrimethamine and is usually successful if started early enough. This needs be continued indefinitely as relapses are common and it is impossible to eradicate toxoplasma gondii completely. These drugs can be given orally or intravenously.

Dementia

Occasionally people with AIDS show signs of forgetfulness, poor concentration and lethargy, and they may behave rather oddly. This form of dementia is normally seen in the later stages of illness but minor signs may appear earlier. Diagnosis is confirmed by the clinical history, psychometric testing, a brain scan to reveal cerebral atrophy and the exclusion of other conditions such as an infection which may cause similar symptoms. Careful, professional diagnosis is essential because symptoms can be similar to those caused by stress, anxiety and depression. The speed at which this disease develops, and its severity, vary. Some people eventually become bedridden and completely dependent on their carers. Some researchers have reported improvements after early symptoms have been treated promptly with zidovudine.

Other neurological symptoms

HIV may affect parts of the nervous system other than the brain. The spinal cord may be affected, resulting in a spastic paraparaesis (weakness/paralysis of the legs), causing difficulty in walking, and may eventually lead to someone being confined to a wheelchair. Investigations are needed to exclude causes other than HIV infection which may be treatable.

Skin

Problems of the skin are numerous and cause additional distress when they are clearly visible on the face or other exposed parts of the body.

Kaposi's sarcoma (KS)

Kaposi's sarcoma is sometimes the first sign of AIDS. It may appear on any part of the skin. It usually first appears as red blotches, which turn into hard, raised, purple lesions. These can appear singly or as multiple lesions on the arms, legs, chest, back, face and neck. KS can also affect the mouth, throat and internal organs such as the gut, lungs and the liver, where it may cause localised symptoms. The clinical course of KS is very variable. Some people develop only a few lesions and suffer no symptoms, while in others the disease spreads and becomes the main cause of death. Treatment depends on the severity of disease and location of lesions. As yet there is no cure so treatment can only relieve symptoms. Single or isolated lesions are not normally treated but if they are on the face where they may cause embarrassment, or if there is any danger that they may affect the throat, local radiotherapy is often used successfully. Counselling may be particularly important here; cosmetic camouflage can also help – see page 75. When KS affects internal organs treatment may be by chemotherapy. This sometimes makes little or no difference. Chemotherapy (treatment with drugs) is normally given as a course over a few days, repeated every few weeks. Close monitoring is needed as side effects such as nausea and vomiting are common. An alternative form of chemotherapy is alpha-interferon. Clinical trials have shown that this has some effect on about 30 per cent of people treated, but high doses can damage the bone marrow. Low-dose alpha-interferon in combination with the drug zidovudine is currently undergoing trials.

Rashes

Some rashes may appear to have no identifiable cause or occasionally be a reaction to the drugs used to treat the various manifestations of AIDS.

Pressure sores

Anyone who spends a long time in bed is liable to develop pressure sores. These develop at pressure points – the places which support your weight as you lie in bed – usually the buttocks, shoulder blades, heels, arms and hips. They can be extremely painful and ugly and can develop into very large open sores which themselves are liable to infection. Pressure sores should be prevented. It is very difficult to cure them after they have developed when someone is bed-bound. They can be prevented by using special mattresses and pads (such as a special rug made of sheepskin), and by ensuring that the person does not lie in the same position for more than a few hours. It may help to massage any red areas which are the first sign of pressure sores. See page 115 for more information.

Herpes

Herpes zoster – shingles – is very common. This consists of a rash formed from multiple blisters which burst and crust over. Shingles can appear anywhere on the skin but is most common on the trunk. It can be very painful, and the pain can remain after the rash has disappeared. Herpes simplex (a virus which causes cold sores and genital ulcers) can also be extremely painful. Salt water baths may relieve the symptoms of ulcers caused by infections of herpes simplex. The drug acyclovir is used to treat both herpes simplex infections and herpes zoster. It works only if it is given early.

Other skin problems

These include minor opportunistic infections such as seborrhoeic dermatitis (appearing as red scaly patches especially on the face, around the nose, and eyebrows and in the scalp) and acne. They are often symptoms of ARC as well as AIDS. Others are tinea (a fungus) and molluscum contagiosum – (small dome-shaped lesions usually on the face and chest, which are not life-threatening and can be easily removed). Dry skin may be helped by using an aqueous cream.

Anti-HIV treatment

The need for an effective anti-HIV drug is urgent. Much research is going on to find a drug that has few side effects, halts the progress of the disease, can be orally absorbed and produced at low cost. The difficulties are immense. So far only one drug, zidovudine, has been licensed. Many others are now under trial.

Zidovudine (formally known as AZT; brand name Retrovir) works by preventing the virus from forming a DNA copy of itself, which in effect stops it reproducing. However, it also affects other processes of the body and so has unpleasant side effects. As the drug doesn't kill the virus but just stops it reproducing it has to be taken indefinitely.

In a major trial in the USA it was shown that zidovudine reduced deaths, decreased the severity and frequency of opportunistic infections and relieved some symptoms. Follow-up of those who took part in this trial showed that after one year only 15 per cent of those who had received it had died – without the drug it was estimated that about half would have died. Unfortunately after two years the survival rate had fallen to 47 per cent.

The major drawback is that between two and four months after the start of treatment it affects the bone marrow of up to half of those treated. (Bone marrow makes blood, and so this leads to anaemia.) This effect reverses itself when the drug is no longer being taken. Blood transfusions may be necessary for some people. Another possible effect is proximal myopathy – a weakness in certain muscles which may, for example, mean that it is more difficult to run, climb stairs or get up from a sitting position. These weaknesses also disappear when AZT is no longer being taken. Nausea and vomiting also occur especially in the first one or two weeks of therapy. These symptoms are normally mild and temporary. Current recommendations are for a dose of 250mg every six hours. Other dosages are being investigated to try and reduce the incidence of toxicity.

Other treatments

Other anti-HIV drugs under test include AL-721, alpha-interferon, ampligen, dextran sulphate, dideoxycytidine, dideoxyinosine and soluble CD4.

One of the most promising seems to be soluble CD4. It mimics the part of the T–helper cell to which HIV attaches itself, causing the virus to bind itself to the CD4 rather than to the cell. Apart from zidovudine and AL721 all other anti-HIV drugs are under test and are available only in clinical trial (see below). AL721 can be obtained on prescription on a compassionate basis under Statutory Instrument No 1450 The Medicines (Exceptions from Licences) (Special and Transitional Cases) Order 1971.

Early intervention

Drugs to prevent specific major opportunistic infections such as PCP (see above) from developing are already given to people who are at risk from them. It is hoped that treatment will be developed for people who are HIV-positive (and without symptoms) which will ward off or prevent the development of ARC or AIDS. At present such treatments are available only as part of trials – see page 196. Developments may include:

- drugs which act on HIV itself – trials to see whether zidovudine is effective are under way (recent trials in the USA have shown that it has been effective for people who have early minor symptoms)
- development of a vaccine to maintain the immune system.

Apart from the fact that early intervention may prove effective, it has the psychological advantage of positive action. On the other hand treatments which do not work can be a waste of energy, be discouraging and a source of further stress. And some drugs could even be harmful.

It is impossible to give any conclusive advice at the moment. It is vital to get as much up-to-date information and advice as you can about the latest results of trials and about what is available – see below.

More information

Information about HIV and its treatment is changing fast. The more information a person with HIV has, the more able he or she will be to talk to doctors and participate in decisions. Choosing what medical treatment to have, if any, may be a matter of thinking about possible risks and possible benefits. However, while your doctor has a duty to tell you something about the suggested treatment, it is up to him or her to decide how much information to give. Doctors are obliged to answer questions so it would be sensible to ask questions about success rates, risks and side effects. It should help to collect as much information as you can in advance.

Organisations who keep up-to-date with the latest thinking and findings of research include Body Positive (page 59), Frontliners (page 60), the Terrence Higgins Trust (page 57), and the Scottish AIDS Monitor (page 58). Centres such as the London Lighthouse (page 67), Kobler Centre (page 66) and Mildmay Mission (page 72) should also be able to help. Also consult your local AIDS helpline. Newsletters published by Body Positive include information on treatment.

FACTS

FACTS (Foundation for AIDS Counselling Treatment and Support) provides medical and other information to doctors, nurses and other medical staff concerned with HIV. They may be able to help you find a good GP, and may be able to help with any problem you have with doctors or other medical professionals. They also have a diagnosis service and can advise GPs on appropriate care following this. Alternatively they can offer a GP-type service themselves for people who are HIV-positive, who don't want their own GP to be involved. Tel. 01-340 6083 (01-348 8809 from mid 1990)

If you want to research things thoroughly yourself, the following publications should help. Your library may suggest where you can borrow a copy.

AIDS Information is a bibliography (with short summaries) of world literature on HIV and AIDS. It is compiled by the Oncology Information Service at the University of Leeds from original papers published in over 1300 biomedical journals. It includes research on treatment, transmission, and social and legal issues, and is published every month. Photocopies of the journals listed can be obtained at 25p a page. *Aids Information* costs £20 to NHS staff/institutions; £40 otherwise. Enquiries to:

Bailey Brothers & Swinfen Ltd
Warner House
Bowles Well Gardens
Folkestone CT19 6PH   (0303) 850501

Current AIDS Literature is a monthly bibliographic service providing an overview of research literature from over 1400 journals on social, biomedical and public health aspects of AIDS. It is produced in association with the Bureau of Hygiene and Tropical Diseases – see below. The Bureau also has a library and database of research articles and other publications on HIV and AIDS.

The subscription in 1990 is £80 (personal); £120 (institutional). Details from:

Current Science Ltd
34–42 Cleveland Street
London W1P 5FB   01-323 0323

Current Science also publish *AIDS*, a monthly journal which includes original papers on clinical and scientific matters, reviews, a bibliography and statistics. The subscription is £60 (personal), £100 (institutional), including an annual review (also available separately – £35 + £5 p+p)

The Lancet and the *British Medical Journal* print articles about medical research into HIV and its treatment. Also useful may be the *New Scientist* and *Scientific American*.

A number of other journals report on developments in treatment. *AIDS Newsletter* contains a synopsis of recent developments. It is aimed at health-care and other professional staff, and costs £45 a year from:

Bureau of Hygiene and Tropical Diseases
Keppel Street
London WC1E 7HT   01-636 8636

AIDS/HIV Experimental Treatment Directory is published four times a year. It gives descriptive (not evaluative) information about current experimental treatments for HIV, AIDS and associated opportunistic infections. Annual subscription: $30 in the USA; $50 elsewhere; single copies $10 in the USA; $15 elsewhere.

American Foundation for AIDS Research
1515 Broadway
Suite 3601
New York NY 10036–8901
USA   Tel. 0101 212 719 0033

AIDS Treatment News reports on experimental and complementary treatments, especially those in current use. The annual subscription (26 issues) is $100 ($150 for organisations); $30 for people with HIV who cannot afford the standard rate (all plus $20 for postage).

ATN Publications
PO Box 411256
San Francisco
CA 94141
USA   Tel. 0101 415 255 0588

For information about these and other journals or sources of information, contact the Terrence Higgins Trust Library (but note that if you want to visit the library you must make an appointment), National or local AIDS helpline or Body Positive.

Trials

You may be asked to take part in a trial of a new medicine or treatment. It is important that you have full information about this, and that your decision is based on a complete understanding of what may be involved. It is up to you whether you participate or not; if you do you will have to sign a consent form. You can withdraw from a trial at any time.

The trial should have been approved by an *ethics committee* which will ensure that the patient's best interests are being respected. If there is no ethics committee get in touch with one of the organisations listed in this chapter. The nature of the trial should be fully explained. You should be told of any possible benefits and of any side effects or drawbacks and given an idea of the level of any risk involved. If you are not given a written summary and explanation of the trial, ask for one so that you can discuss it with someone you trust.

Many people agree to take part in tests because of the chance that an experimental or new treatment or drug will work. However many trials are made with a *control*. This means that some of the people selected for a trial are given a *placebo* rather than the new treatment – this is a harmless substance which looks like the drug being tested. This is done so that the effects of the drug can be compared to what would happen if it wasn't used. Using a placebo means that any effect due to people getting better because they think they are getting treatment is allowed for. In such tests you will not know whether you have been given the real drug or the placebo. Often the doctor carrying out the test will not know either.

You should ask the doctor if the trial will include placebos. However, there is little you can do to make sure you are being treated with the drug being tested rather than being part of the control group. Some people argue that there is no need for placebo tests because the effects of not treating HIV infection are already well known. People who have developed ARC or AIDS are unlikely to be asked to take part in trials involving a placebo, because treatment with zidovudine is known to be effective and it would be unethical to stop anyone taking it. If future trials with asymptomatic patients are successful, placebo controls may become unethical for this group, too.

11 *Complementary medicine*

Doctors in Western countries are trained in allopathic (that is to say orthodox or conventional) medicine. Very broadly, this considers that illness occurs when the normal balance of the body is upset by outside influences – viruses, bacteria, physical damage, poison and so on. Diseases are generally treated by surgery or chemicals.

Complementary therapies also may treat the immediate causes of symptoms, or even the symptoms themselves. But they often place emphasis on preventive maintenance of the body. Treatment is usually aimed at finding and correcting ways in which the body is in conflict with its environment – including emotional stresses caused by frustration and anxiety. Complementary therapies are often referred to as holistic or wholistic medicine because of their concern for all aspects of a person's life rather than with a particular illness. Many therapies involve combinations of positive thought, good nutrition, regular exercise and stress reduction, all of which are likely to be beneficial in their own right.

Some people with HIV have found complementary medicine has helped them stay healthy. There is an enormous range of therapies to choose from. These include well-established treatments such as homeopathy, acupuncture and massage, systems of relaxation and stress reduction such as autogenic training. In addition, there are therapies and organisations which focus on HIV – these offer, for example, classes in 'AIDS Mastery', spiritual approaches to healing, courses of nutrition including special dietary products such as AL-721 ('egg yolk' therapy).

The evidence in favour of any particular complementary therapy is likely to be based on individual case histories and practitioners' assessments of their own success rate. Scientific, comparative trials are difficult and, some would argue, inappropriate. Very few have been tested in controlled experiments. It is difficult to know if the successes claimed are due to the therapy, to chance, or to a placebo effect (getting better because you expect to). This is not to say that the therapies don't work, just that you shouldn't expect to find conclusive scientific evidence one way or the other. Our advice is to be very cautious – anyone considering a complementary therapy should find out as much as possible about any therapy they feel an affinity for before going ahead.

The Terrence Higgins Trust library can supply information about journals which may have up-to-date information about recent trials.

The British Library, jointly with the Research Council for Complementary Medicine, produce a monthly literature bulletin, *Complementary Medicine Index*, and will give information about published and unpublished research. See also sources of information given on page 193.

British Library Medical Information Service
Boston Spa
Wetherby
West Yorkshire LS23 7BQ   (0937) 843434

Finding a practitioner

One of the main problems is finding a good practitioner.

Many organisations award diplomas, membership of professional bodies and even degrees. Some require little medical knowledge, and some training, considering the range of ailments practitioners may treat, can be superficial. The diplomas and documents a practitioner may have on display may not be a guide to his or her merit.

The Institute for Complementary Medicine exists to publicise the practice of complementary remedies and keeps tabs on what the different diplomas mean. Through a network of local information officers they can put you in touch with practitioners who meet certain standards – for example, belonging to a professional organisation which has a Code of Practice, having liability and accident insurance. To find your nearest information officer, send an SAE to:

Information Office
Institute for Complementary Medicine
21 Portland Place
London W1N 3AF   01-636 9543

HART

The Holistic AIDS Research Trust (HART) is an information service which aims to encourage research and provide information about 'alternative, complementary and self-help techniques' and their practitioners.

BM HART
London WC1N 3XX   (0273) 698698

Local doctors may also know what's available in your area. Your local AIDS helpline may also have information about local groups, workshops and courses.

London Lighthouse (see page 67) have courses on different holistic approaches to health and on particular therapies, including 'taster' sessions which provide an opportunity to try out a number of different therapies.

Before you choose a particular therapy find out about the range available – it may be that the first one you hear of isn't the most suitable. If you can, speak to people who have been treated by the therapist you are thinking of going to. Find out if he or she has worked with people with HIV-related diseases before. Remember to check beforehand how much a course of therapy or treatment is likely to cost. And also bear in mind that complementary therapy is just that – it doesn't mean that you have to turn your back on conventional medicine or restrict yourself to one alternative therapy. According to the *National AIDS Manual* a flexible 'cocktail' of therapies works best for many people with HIV. Once you have started a course, monitor your progress. Don't expect immediate results but maintain a keen awareness of whether it is doing any good or not.

12

Partners and families

In this section we look at some of the special situations faced when caring for a partner and caring for a relative.

Caring for a partner

Taking the test

If the person with AIDS is your partner you may also be concerned about your own health. There is a possibility that you may be HIV-positive yourself. It is important that you have some way of discussing your feelings about this, either with your partner or someone else. If you want to be tested it may be better to do this fairly soon. Some carers who have found out they were HIV-positive at a time when their partner was very ill have been afraid to further burden their partner with the news. This can be a tremendously stressful situation. Some people avoid having a test to prevent this situation arising.

There are many things to take into account before deciding to have a test. There are practical considerations concerning insurance and endowment mortgages (see page 95). More fundamental are the emotional consequences of a positive result. Some people feel they could not cope with 'knowing'. They argue that if they are already practising safer sex and being sensible about diet and exercise there is nothing more they could be doing, and being told that they are HIV-positive would just add another layer of stress to their lives – a positive test result doesn't mean you will develop AIDS or even minor infections. Other people find the uncertainty of not knowing stressful in itself and wish to settle the matter one way or the other, particularly if they begin to worry at the onset of every minor illness or begin to imagine symptoms.

Before you finally decide, think about how you would feel and what you would do if the result turned out to be *positive*. Some people find it helpful to talk around this situation until they are clear about what they want to do. Once you have taken the test there is no going back so you need to be sure of yourself.

Although no one knows what therapies may be developed in the future to combat HIV infection, there is no cure at present. Some people believe that as nothing can be done there is little point in the test. The only real precautions you need to take concern safer sex. But you should be doing this anyway, irrespective of the results of the test. If you are HIV-positive you have the responsibility of protecting others from infection. If you are not you should be taking the same precautions to protect yourself. However, if you are actually ill and a doctor experienced in the field feels that the results of the test would affect treatment for the illness you would be well advised to take it. Similarly, it may be sensible to have one if you think you could be HIV-positive and want to get pregnant – see page 213.

You also may need to know your HIV status if you need a vaccination. If you are HIV-positive you may need different doses or special vaccines. Before having a vaccination you should tell the doctor that you are HIV-positive. Department of Health guidelines state that live vaccines for measles, mumps, rubella and polio are safe for people with an HIV infection (although those who have *symptoms* of an HIV-related illness may be given an inactivated form of polio vaccine). Inactivated vaccines for whooping cough, diphtheria, tetanus, cholera and hepatitis B are also safe. There is no risk from malaria tablets. People who are HIV-positive should not be given BCG vaccine (for TB). Injections for yellow fever should not be given to people who are HIV-positive and have the symptoms of an HIV-related illness. Those who are HIV-positive but have no symptoms should check with their GP.

If you do decide to take a test, contact your local AIDS advice service to find a trained counsellor who can advise you.

Sex

Both you and your partner may have fears about transmitting HIV during sex. Even if you are both HIV-positive the general advice is to keep to safer sex practices – see Appendices. If you spend time at this point on the physical aspects of your relationship it will help to avoid problems later. Although it is hard at first to change long standing sexual behaviour it is possible to do so without reducing intimacy, physical closeness or erotic pleasure. Many people have reported increased sexual enjoyment, probably as a direct result of a new emotional closeness.

Soon after being diagnosed HIV-positive, however, your partner might not feel like having any sexual contact at all. This may be due to fears of infecting you, a lower self–image or because of a genuine loss of libido. It is easy for any changes at this time to be misinterpreted. It is therefore vital to discuss them. Your partner may need enormous amounts of reassurance that he or she has not suddenly become undesirable. It is very important for you not to feel rejected because your partner has seemed to turn away. It is far more likely to indicate a fear of rejection.

I find I have to handle the relationship with kid gloves because his big hang-up is that he will infect me. For a long time I was not allowed to touch him at all or kiss and the fear of sex turned him off any form of physical contact

Occasionally the fear and disinclination for continuation of the sexual side of the relationship cannot be overcome. This does not mean that the relationship is over. Groups such as Frontliners (page 60), Body Positive (page 59), Positive Partners (page 61) and others described in this book will be able to arrange for counselling if you decide this will help. Generally the more specialised the group and the more attuned they are to your situation, the better.

Albany Trust

General advice on sexual and associated psychological problems and problems with relationships is also given by the Albany Trust. Counselling can be individual or in groups. They charge £18–£20 for the initial interview, although this and fees for subsequent sessions can be negotiated. If you cannot afford to pay, you will not be turned away.

Albany Trust Counselling
24 Chester Square
London SW1W 9HS   01-730 5871

SPOD

SPOD (Sexual and Personal Relationships of People with a Disability) was set up to help those with sexual difficulties relating to disability. However, they also have an uninhibited counselling service and will be pleased to talk to anyone with AIDS or affected by HIV.

> SPOD
> 286 Camden Road
> London N7 OBJ   01-607 8851

Pressure on the relationship

The needs of partners often go unrecognised. The trauma of living with AIDS can obviously put an enormous pressure on the most secure relationship. In these circumstances couples tend either to realise how much they care for each other and so become much closer – or grow apart. Previous problems in the relationship can be exaggerated by AIDS to the extent that the relationship ends. This can be heartbreaking. Sometimes, if HIV prompts someone to end a poor or deteriorating relationship, this can be a positive step.

Your partner may have acquired the virus through sexual contact with a third party. This may be a painful issue to face, but, according to research carried out in London, does not usually lead to people separating. However, some agreement might have to be reached about future contacts with others. Clear expression of feeling on both sides is crucial – now as later.

Another common problem is when the roles of each partner changes. One partner may have to bear the responsibility of all domestic and practical tasks, or may begin to take decisions which would previously have been shared or have been dealt with by the other partner. Someone who was once fiercely independent may suddenly find he or she has to rely on someone else. Some relationships do not survive these changes.

There are special difficulties where both partners are infected but only one is ill. The well partner may see what is happening to the other as a prediction of the future. This can be a good thing when the partner is coping well and the illness is associated with some positive experiences. However, if it is unpleasant or painful, the effect on the well partner can be devastating. Talking through fears will help, and it is important to hang on to the fact that being HIV-positive does not necessarily mean that ARC or AIDS will follow, and that ways of managing and containing associated illnesses are improving all the time. Surprisingly, perhaps, communication can be a problem. Either partner may decide not to talk too much about the illness or share his or her own distress for fear of worrying the other. Often this silence may cause more worry than open discussion. Some people may have problems expressing their feelings about the illness, or be so uncertain about it that sounding sensible becomes difficult.

You have to build on what you have in a relationship rather than be aware of what is no longer possible. Think about the things you can share – talking, listening to music, touching. Many people with AIDS and their partners have reported that many of the changes in their relationships have been positive. HIV has had an integrating and stabilising effect on some relationships, especially when people spend more time together communicating, planning, or spending time on activities which would normally go by the board. Very often couples become both mentally and physically closer.

Gay partners

The problems discussed above can apply to anyone, gay or straight. Gay partners may have additional difficulties. While some people do not meet any prejudice, and manage to be very open about their relationship and about HIV, others have very great problems. The problems of keeping things secret can be immense, particularly in small communities and especially if you need to involve local helping agencies. Your local AIDS helpline may be able to help with advice and information about local services known to be particularly discreet.

It can be difficult to explain why you need to take time off work. It can be impossible to show grief or talk about your concerns. This cuts you off from a lot of support and sympathy, and not sharing such an important part of your life can mean that your relationships with casual friends or workmates are cooler than they would be otherwise.

There have been extreme cases where people have been ostracised or have become a target of abuse. This is extremely difficult to deal with. Some people have been affected by discrimination to an extent that their own view of themselves is lowered. Some people feel guilt about HIV or even about being gay.

The befriending, counselling and support services described in this book are particularly important in these circumstances, and support groups of other partners or carers will be invaluable.

Families

The issues that arise for family members will depend on the nature of the relationship before HIV was diagnosed. As a family member you may find you are facing things inherited from the past as well as the current situation. There is a possibility that old conflicts may be rekindled. Some family members may not be told until quite late on that their relative has AIDS. Generally speaking those that are closest are told soonest. Many find it difficult to cope with the shock.

Families are often dispersed across the country. This makes it much more difficult for them to offer support without causing additional problems. Do you drive 200 miles to stay for a cup of tea, or do you stay a week? The only way these questions can be answered is by careful consideration after talking to the person with AIDS and the other people involved.

It is very important that you do not disturb existing sources of support. Some parents have not been able to accept their son's lover as the main carer and have caused great disruption. Bear in mind, too, that it is possible to help too much, which can mean that the person with AIDS becomes passive or that he or she becomes busy trying to find things for you to do in the belief that it is keeping you happy or helping you deal with the situation.

Dealing with the emotional upheaval can also put pressure on the parents' relationship itself. Parents are also likely to feel isolated. It is difficult to talk openly about one's feelings because of fears of prejudice. Many parents keep the details of the diagnosis within the family, perhaps claiming that their son or daughter has cancer.

Families may also have to face their own fears, prejudices and misconceptions at this point. These may be about a son being gay and what they might imagine about his lifestyle. If they discover that a son is gay and has HIV at the same time, this can require a tremendous amount of readjustment. The best way of confronting prejudice may be through information, and through talking to people who have been through similar experiences. It may also help you work out what you can best do to help.

Prejudice and sexuality

Some people don't feel happy about the sexuality of a gay friend or relative. If this applies to you, it may help to think about the following points.

Try to work out what it is that you don't like. The person won't have changed, so why should your attitude be any different? You may be upset because you have not been told before. You have a right to feel upset about this, but try to understand why you haven't been told. Perhaps the person was afraid of your reaction and didn't want to lose you. Maybe the person has experienced bad reactions in the past (most gay people have been called names at some point and can become very sensitive about this). Maybe you have been heard to make comments about gay people and not been told because of this.

If you are a parent you may feel that it is in some way your fault. But why should blame come into it at all? But no one knows what makes people gay, and it is certainly not something to be ashamed of. Try to meet your son's friends – it may help you realise that being gay is something you can feel fine about. You may find the idea of a gay life-style distasteful or disgusting. These feelings will be very powerful and difficult to deal with. The key to getting past them is to be aware that you like and love the person enough to accept his way of life. But if you can't let the person be himself it is probably better to stay away altogether. He will need your support, not your criticism.

You may have fixed ideas about what makes a good or bad relationship. For example, you may feel that a relationship in which one or both partners have sex outside it is lacking in some way. These ideas may be wrong – all relationships are different and what is important is what the couple themselves want out of it. If you are a parent it is quite normal not to be entirely in sympathy with the way your children live their lives, gay or straight. You are both entitled to your views but you have to respect each other's choices.

The reactions of friends or other relatives may hurt you. They may even remind you of feelings you have been trying to overcome. This is their problem rather than yours. However, in practice people may take the cue from your own attitude; if you are at ease the likelihood is that they will become so, too. If you show that someone being gay has not made any difference to your love, they may be able to change too. Many people do have problems of adjustment and these feelings are perfectly understandable. It may help to talk to someone on a Lesbian and Gay Switchboard, with whom you can be free and open. The London

Lesbian and Gay Switchboard (see page 107) will have local telephone numbers. Some groups have been set up to help those coming to terms with the sexuality of relatives or friends.

Acceptance

Acceptance was set up by parents of lesbians and gay men to provide support for other parents. Help is mostly given by telephone but monthly meetings are also held at the house of one family in Kent. They publish a newsletter. Send a 9 inch × 7 inch SAE for information.

If you want someone to talk to, ring (0795) 661463 from 7pm to 9pm, Tuesdays to Fridays.

> Acceptance
> 64 Holmside Avenue
> Halfway Houses
> Sheerness
> Kent ME12 3EY

Positive Partners – see page 61.

Parents' Enquiry

Parents' Enquiry is a counselling service which operates by telephone, by post and on a personal basis for young people who think they may be lesbian or gay, and their families. They publish two pamphlets, *What is Homosexuality?* (mainly for parents and families) and *Telling your Parents* (for young people). There are two trained counsellors and a number of befrienders who will, when necessary, travel to clients' homes for family sessions. No fees are charged, but donations towards postage, telephone and travel costs are welcome.

> Parents' Enquiry
> 16 Honley Road
> Catford
> London SE6 2HZ   01-698 1815 (or 01-788 7512)

Groups such as The Family Support Network (see page 277), Positive Partners (see page 61), and other self-help groups described in chapter 3 will also be able to help.

Sharing a household

There are no special risks from living with someone who is HIV-positive or who has AIDS. You can get HIV infection only if large amounts of the virus manage to get into your bloodstream – see chapter 1. So there is no risk of infection in ordinary domestic situations.

Good standards of household hygiene should be maintained *anyway* as protection from ordinary germs. Advice about hygiene tends to be ultra-cautious to protect against all conceivable eventualities, not just HIV. Remember that the most serious risk is to the person with HIV, for whom picking up an ordinary infection can have serious consequences.

- Wear rubber gloves to clean up spillages of blood, semen, vomit or excrement in case you have cuts on your hands. It's best if these are cleaned up by the person who made them. Use disposable paper which can be flushed down the toilet. Disinfect the areas affected afterwards.
- Use the hot cycle in the washing machine for dirty fabrics.
- Wash cuts well with running water. Let them bleed a little to get rid of any germs. Use an antiseptic to clean the cut and a waterproof plaster to cover it.
- Don't share toothbrushes or razors. There is a tiny theoretical risk of passing on traces of blood, or germs.
- Use very hot water for washing up and different cloths for cleaning the kitchen and bathroom.
- Use gloves when gardening and when handling pets and litter trays.

13 Pregnancy and children

Pregnancy

If one partner is infected with HIV he or she can pass on the infection during unprotected sexual intercourse. Some couples may decide that the risk of infection makes it unwise to start a family. It has been suggested that the actual process of having a baby may increase the risk of an HIV-positive woman developing ARC or AIDS, but there is no conclusive evidence to support this.

If only the man is infected, attempting to have a child carries a double risk of infecting the woman and perhaps the baby. However, in these circumstances a woman may feel that she would like to have a child in case she loses her partner. On the other hand the demands of a pregnancy might make it harder for her to give him the support and care he may need if AIDS develops. There are unfortunately no definite guidelines we can give. All we can suggest is:

- Take advice from experts. Knowledge in this area is constantly changing.
- Take enough time to consider your decision.
- Make sure that you are both agreed about the decision you come to.
- If you decide to go ahead, ensure that you have full medical supervision from the first weeks of your pregnancy.

Check with the doctor at your clinic for the latest assessment of the risks of pregnancy. Or contact Avert (page 222), the Health Education Authority, the Terrence Higgins Trust (page 57) or the Screening Clinic, City Hospital, Edinburgh.

How do children become infected?

About four-fifths of children who have HIV infection acquired it from their mother during her pregnancy. Others have been infected through receiving contaminated blood or blood products (a negligible risk nowadays). Isolated cases of infection have been reported following sexual abuse. The risks of infecting an unborn infant are now thought to vary according to the mother's state of health. Early estimates, based on preliminary reports from a European study, suggest that HIV-positive women who have *no* symptoms of any HIV-related disease may have a one in five chance of infecting a child. Mothers who have the symptoms of HIV disease carry a much greater risk.

It is now thought unlikely that children could be infected during birth, and so decisions about the mode of delivery for HIV-positive women should be taken on the same basis as for anyone else. Extra precautions may be taken at the hospital during the birth to prevent nursing and medical staff becoming infected.

There have been some reports of infection through breast milk but the evidence is not conclusive, and the risk is probably low. Check with the doctor at your clinic about this. Some HIV-positive women decide not to breastfeed, while others feel that the benefits to the baby outweigh the risks. The advantages of breastfeeding, such as balanced nutrition and the emotional benefit to both mother and child, are well known. If a child has been infected by HIV, breastfeeding may help prevent other potentially serious infections. There are no reported cases of children becoming infected at nurseries, playgroups, school, or from normal household contact with someone who is HIV-positive.

Testing children for HIV infection

Children born to women who are HIV-positive are often called 'children at risk of HIV infection'. With current tests it is not possible to know whether a baby born to an HIV-positive mother and still under the age of two has been infected. The reason for this is that the mother's HIV antibodies will be found in the baby's blood. These maternal antibodies will usually disappear at around the time of the baby's first birthday, although there have been cases where antibodies persist until 22 months. So a positive antibody test result before that time doesn't necessarily mean that the baby is infected. If the baby is infected, he or she may begin to make his or her own antibodies, and will therefore continue to test positive. However, if the virus has damaged the immune system, some infected babies may never produce antibodies. A negative result does not therefore necessarily rule out infection. New tests are currently being developed which may help to end this uncertainty for parents and children.

Symptoms

Like adults, children can be infected but remain totally well. Little is known about them because they have never needed medical treatment. As with adults it is difficult to generalise about the ways in which the disease may show itself or develop. There is no set pattern and early signs do not necessarily mean that children may go on to develop AIDS.

Some affected children have shown a slower physical or mental development than average. This can affect walking or control of limbs and can result in seizures. It is thought that children with neurological problems may be helped with the drug zidovudine. Some children have developed problems with their lungs and some more severe cases have needed long-term oxygen therapy. Other symptoms have been secondary cancers, such as lymphoma of the central nervous system. HIV is also reported to have affected the heart, kidneys and liver.

In the early stages of HIV disease, children may show signs and symptoms which are quite common in children without HIV infection. Examples of these are diarrhoea, runny nose, sore ears, sore throat, skin rashes, fevers and chest infections. Many children are slow to put on weight.

Caring for children

For people caring for an HIV-positive child there is constant anxiety about the child's health. It is hard to know whether you should worry about every trivial symptom, which may be just a childhood ailment or the sign of an HIV-related disease. In either case medical advice is important – prompt treatment of minor infections may be helpful in preventing further difficulties. Early recognition of patterns of infection may be useful in working out future treatment. You should not feel that you have been left with the responsibility of assessing the significance of symptoms alone; make sure you get as much help and reassurance as possible.

An HIV-positive child should be allowed to live a normal life, should attend school and take part in the usual activities of his or her age group. Good hygiene practice at home is enough to prevent the spread of non-sexual infection. As a rule live vaccines are safe apart from BCG vaccine, but consult your doctor about this. See page 204 for more information about vaccines.

Should you tell anyone if a child is HIV-positive?

There are no easy answers to this difficult question. A couple of points worth thinking about are: who has the *right* to know and who *needs* to know? It may be that no one has the right to know, but that there are some people whom the parents feel they would like to tell. Some families feel that only those people who *have* to know should know; but who those people are will be different in every case. Clearly the child's family doctor and health visitor should know as they need to provide appropriate health care, and will be involved in day-to-day care, treatment and support for the parents or carers of the child.

People also need support from within their own circle. You may have friends or relatives who would offer support if they were aware of the need for it. However, it is worth taking time to think about how each person might react. Some people may be totally unreasonably worried about the risk of transmission. A balance needs to be struck between the need for support and help, and the risk of a hurtful and damaging rejection by others. Some families find it helpful to think through the whole subject of whom to tell (and when) with a counsellor.

The task of keeping the infection a secret may be burdensome or even impossible. A few families have decided they should be completely open from the beginning. Some families report that this was, for them, the only choice and have no regrets about it. Others have found that local people have reacted very badly and they have been treated very harshly as a result. Each family will need to find its own way through this very difficult area, and most families do seem to be able to work out a solution. Remember that if you do tell, there is no going back.

Babysitters and child-minders

Some parents or carers believe they should tell babysitters or childminders about the child's infection; others disagree.

Ordinary good hygiene is enough to prevent transmission of the virus, even when body fluids are spilled. People who are confident that good hygiene would be practised anyway may decide not to tell. Others are uncomfortable about this, particularly if there is any likelihood that the babysitter or childminder might find out later. It is also important to think about the risks of other children or adults passing on an infection such as chickenpox to the child. You do not have to tell a childminder that any special concerns you have about this are because of HIV, of course.

Playgroups, nurseries and schools

In England and Wales, the Department of Education and Science and, in Scotland, the Scottish Education Department, have advised local authorities that there is no necessity for parents to inform schools or nurseries if a child is HIV-positive as normal good hygiene practice is sufficient to prevent infection. Also, if staff rely on knowing who is infected and who isn't, they may be selective in their hygiene, and expose themselves and others in situations where they do not believe they are at risk. Everyone is safer when care is taken all the time. Schools in particular should be practising good hygiene anyway to protect children against such infections as hepatitis B and meningitis.

However, some people feel that it is in the child's interest to tell staff that your child is HIV-positive – for example, if it would help staff give a child additional care or consideration. It may even be possible, although very difficult, for the child's infection not to be referred to by name. Once again, careful thought must be given to the possible effects of sharing the information.

At school, the only documented risk to HIV-positive children whose immune system has been damaged is that of being more likely to catch illnesses, such as measles or chickenpox. It may be necessary to keep them away temporarily when such potentially serious illnesses are around. No special risks are involved in school activities such as sharing wind instruments, sports and home economics classes for which normal hygienic practices are observed. Special thought should be given if children have widespread open skin lesions, or are behaviourally disturbed, or developmentally delayed. In such circumstances you should always get medical advice. Children should be discouraged from becoming 'blood' brothers or sisters, in which blood is shared as a kind of bond. Ear piercing and tattooing is safe only if properly sterilised needles are used. The Department of Education and Science have two free leaflets – see page 222.

Talking to children about HIV

Views vary about the amount a child should be told about his or her own illness. Generally, children respond better to information which is given to them sensitively, in a form they can understand and by someone they trust. The child's age and ability to understand what is being said are therefore the most important considerations. Children under the age of eight have very limited appreciation of what death means, though they do understand illness. It will not be possible to explain everything at once so it would be best to see it as a task for a number of conversations. Once the subject has been broached, give the child opportunities to ask questions about what has been said, and add new pieces of information gradually. More questions will follow very quickly, giving you the chance to explain further. Knowing that you have an infection that may bring about your death is very frightening, so it is important to give a child plenty of opportunities to express fears and sadness.

Children and sex education

Children who are HIV-positive, whether they have symptoms or not, will need to be aware of their own sexuality, and understand the nature of sexual relationships before they will be able to appreciate what their own infection means. Often children begin their sexual explorations earlier than those caring for them expect, and it is important that you help them understand how the virus is transmitted so that they do not expose others to risk. Sexual awareness in children is a difficult subject for many adults to deal with, and some feel unable to cope with it at all, or believe they will do it badly. Where there are further complications of a sexually transmissible infection, the topic may become even more difficult and painful, particularly as it may be necessary to discuss safer sex with young people who have little or no experience, and who are still learning about their bodies, their emotions and their relationships. Parents and young people may well find it particularly helpful to get outside advice and support in tackling sex and safer sex education – see pages 91 and 221.

Some parents will feel that they were responsible for their child's illness. It is important to try to separate the feelings of sadness about the child's illness and possible death from any feelings of guilt, which would prevent you helping the child as much as possible. Obviously parents are uniquely important to children, and the way in which they deal with the child's condition will be a cornerstone in the child's own way of coping. Two useful books which help children to talk about death are *Badger's Parting Gifts* by Susan Varley (Collins), £1.95; *When Uncle Bob Died* by Althea (Dinosaur), £1.75. You should feel free to solicit advice and support from wherever it can be best given – whether in helping a child to understand the situation, in making decisions about treatment or in the handling of relationships. Your local AIDS information line or treatment clinic may be able to put you in touch with appropriate services. Also see the section on counselling on page 83, and details of organisations on page 85.

Care and guardianship

Compulsory care

Some parents worry about the powers their local authority has to take children into care compulsorily. In *England and Wales* this can happen only if the local authority is concerned about the child's welfare. The fact that a parent or parents have an HIV infection or AIDS would *not* be sufficient, in itself, for a local authority to seek to take a child into care.

To take a child into care without the consent of the parent(s) the local authority would need to make an application to a court for a care order. At present some of the grounds for this are when a child is out of control or in moral danger; when his or her development is being avoidably neglected or prevented; when health is being avoidably impaired; or when a violent or sexual offence has been committed against the child by a member of the same household. In each case the court would also have to be satisfied that the child was in need of care or control which he or she would not get unless an order were made.

If it appears to the court that there is, or may be, a conflict of interests between the child and the parent(s), the parent(s) may be made party to the proceedings. In this case, parents may be legally represented if they wish, and are entitled to apply for Legal Aid. They may also appeal against the decision of the Court.

The Children Bill currently being discussed in Parliament may change this situation. It proposes that children may be taken into care if they have suffered, or are likely to suffer, significant harm because of an unreasonably low standard of care or because the child is beyond parental control. The court would have to be convinced that the care order was in the child's best interests and that making an order would be better for the child than not making one (i.e. that the local authority can do better than the parents). The Bill covers England and Wales.

In Scotland, anyone may refer a child to the Reporter of the *Children's Panel* on the grounds that he or she may be in need of compulsory measures of care. However, the Reporter will arrange for the child to appear before a children's hearing only if he or she considers that there are sufficient grounds for considering that compulsory measures of care may be necessary. Among the grounds for this are when a child is beyond the parents' control or is falling into bad associations or is exposed to moral danger; when lack of parental care is likely to cause unnecessary suffering or seriously impair health or development; when a violent or sexual offence has been committed against a child by a member of the same household; when a child has failed to attend school regularly without a reasonable excuse, or when a child has committed an offence.

The grounds for referral to the hearing must be accepted by the child and parent(s) for the case to proceed. If they are not accepted, or the child is too young to understand the grounds, then the case may be referred to the Sheriff Court. If the Sheriff finds the grounds proved, the case goes back to the hearing for the Panel to decide what to do. If the Sheriff finds the grounds not proved, the case is dismissed. (If the child is under the age of eight, or if the parent or child disagrees with the grounds of the referral, the case is heard in the Sheriff Court.)

Legal Aid is not available for appearances before a children's hearing, but may be available if the case is referred to the Sheriff Court. The child or parent(s) may appeal to the Sheriff Court against the decision of a hearing and again Legal Aid may be available for this purpose.

Voluntary care

A local authority may also be able to provide facilities for voluntary care. This is given at the request of a parent or guardian when temporary help is needed in caring for the child. This might be particularly important for parents who are ill, at times when they are unable to care for their child, or when they need a rest. In these circumstances, you should approach your local authority social services department or, in Scotland, the social work department.

Guardianship

If parents themselves are ill it would be sensible to consider who would look after and bring up their child in the event of their deaths. It is possible to make provision in a will for a testamentary guardian – someone chosen to care for a child following the death of the parents. The child would then be brought up in the way the parents would prefer and this may also avoid legal and family difficulties which might arise if no provision is made. This is an important decision, and one which should be given a great deal of thought. Parents may want a guardian who is young enough to be an active parent, and whose views on parenting and child care are similar to their own. Having decided who would be the best person, it is essential to discuss it extremely thoroughly with him or her, and then inform other family members who may have an interest in the child's future. This would provide an opportunity to explain the decision and may prevent feelings being hurt later.

Help and advice

Children with HIV may need any of the ordinary services available to children, or they may need special services set up to help with HIV. As a rule the best place to go to discuss a child's needs would be the social services department – see page 53. Many departments have begun to train their staff to deal with the problems associated with HIV, and carers such as foster parents, residential staff and nursery staff may be able to help.

The Terrence Higgins Trust (page 57), the Haemophilia Society (page 246) and London Lighthouse (page 67) will be able to give information and advice on children. Also contact your local AIDS helpline. NAYPCAS (page 91) will be able to give information about counselling *for* young people.

Positively Women

Positively Women is a self-help group for women who are HIV-positive or who have ARC or AIDS. They will give advice, face-to-face counselling and have a support group in London.

Positively Women
333 Gray's Inn Road
London WC1X 8PX   01-837 9705

Positive Women in Scotland

Positive Women in Scotland (not part of Positively Women) is only for women who are HIV-positive or who have ARC or AIDS. It gives practical help (such as babysitting or assistance with applications for grants) and holds meetings and one-to-one 'listening sessions', either over the phone or face to face.

> 37–39 Montrose Terrace
> Edinburgh EH7 5DJ   031-652 0754

AVERT

AVERT will be able to tell you where to go for more information, and counselling support on HIV and pregnancy, as well as other matters relating to women and children.

> AVERT (Aids Education and Research Trust)
> PO Box 91
> Horsham
> West Sussex RH13 7YR   (0403) 864010

Department of Education and Science

Children at School and Problems Related to AIDS, which is available free from: DES, Publications Despatch Centre, Canons Park HA7 1AZ and Welsh Office, Information Division, Cathays Park, Cardiff CF1 3NQ (Welsh language version available on request).

AIDS: Some Questions and Answers Facts for Teachers, Lecturers and Youth Workers, which is available free from the address above, and Scottish Education Department, New St Andrew's House, St James Centre, Edinburgh EH1 3SY and Department of Education, Northern Ireland, Rathgael House, Balloo Road, Bangor, Co Down BT19 2PR.

National Childbirth Trust

The National Childbirth Trust (NCT) offer ante-natal and post-natal support. They also publish leaflets and books about pregnancy, birth, breastfeeding and parenthood. There are over 300 local branches and groups in the UK. Full membership costs £15 (£12 for renewal), or you can be a local member. Contact:

> NCT
> Alexandra House
> Oldham Terrace
> London W3 6NH   01-992 8637

National Childminding Association	The National Childminding Association publish a leaflet, *Who Minds about AIDS?*, which has useful information for parent, babysitters and childminders. Single copies are free (25p per copy for bulk orders).

National Childminding Association
8 Masons Hill
Bromley BR2 9EY   01–464 6164

National Foster Care Association

The National Foster Care Association produce a booklet for carers, *Aids and HIV – Information for Foster Parents*, which covers things that need to be considered when caring for other people's children. It costs 80p for non-members, 40p for NFCA members.

National Foster Care Association
Francis House
Francis Street
London SW1P 1DE   01–828 6266

The Voluntary Council for Handicapped Children

The Voluntary Council for Handicapped Children is a consortium of voluntary and professional organisations with a broad interest in children with disability, illness and special needs. It has an extensive information service (leaflets, publications and information on local services).

The Voluntary Council for Handicapped Children
8 Wakley Street
London EC1V 7QE   01–278 9441

Helpful book

The Implications of AIDS for Children in Care, by Daphne Batty, British Agencies for Adoption and Fostering, London 1987.

14

Drugs users and HIV

Using drugs in itself carries no risk of HIV infection. Injecting drug users are at risk if they share needles or have done so in the past. And any kind of drug (including alcohol) can lower inhibitions and may mean that people cease to be careful about safer sex.

This chapter gives information about specialist sources of help for people who are worried about their own or another person's use of drugs. Don't assume that the information in this chapter will apply to all drug users – many use drugs in a controlled way and need no special help or support at all.

Drug users are often wrongly believed to be desperate and violent people who lie, who don't care about themselves and who are likely to hurt anyone who tries to help or love them. This stereotype has meant that many of us brand drug users as criminals, and just shut them out. It makes it difficult, or even impossible, for them to ask for help when they may need it. It forces many of them into hiding and means that they can end up treating any offer of help with the utmost suspicion. Yet, because of their general lifestyles, HIV-positive drug users are probably more at risk of developing ARC or AIDS earlier, and may have more infections. They may face tougher problems, too.

If caring for someone with AIDS brings you into contact with a drug user you don't know, you may have to overcome various fears and even some prejudices. Common, and usually unfounded, worries are about the possibility of violence, theft, and manipulation in an effort to obtain drugs or money for drugs. Lack of sleep, bad diet and poor living conditions can contribute to a person being edgy, which is the way some drug users seem, but experienced workers can cope with this without particular difficulty.

This chapter outlines some points you may have to consider and describes sources of help.

People who use drugs may be intoxicated some of the time. However, you should remember that most remain perfectly capable of sorting out their own problems if they are supported, well advised and given encouragement to do so. Your job as a carer may be to help fill in gaps by providing information, arranging access to health care, finding out about local services or providing some direct care yourself – in short, supplying the knowledge and means for the person you are working with to stay as healthy as possible. What you actually do should depend on the wishes and needs of the person you are caring for, and on the help that you are willing to give.

Some basic guidelines

Use of drugs

Many carers have said that the first hurdle they have had to overcome has been learning to accept the use of drugs rather than to take a censorious line over it. You need to concentrate on the needs of the person rather than on their use of drugs.

It is not your job to pressurise or coerce the person you are caring for into giving up drugs. This is not your choice but theirs. You should respect this right even if you do not agree with what they are doing. Be wary of suggesting treatment unless you are sure you are the right person to begin this discussion. Drug users are used to people trying to persuade them to stop, often without regard to the anguish of doing so, or without any offer of help and support. If you do the same you are likely to be bracketed with previous unsympathetic 'helpers' and this will put a barrier between you and the person. Your first aim must be to build an honest and open relationship, with trust existing on both sides.

A course of treatment will be successful only if the person is motivated enough to complete it. Most drug users eventually do decide to stop using them, and you should accept that this is a goal to be attempted only when the time is right. The person may not have reached the point of wishing to stop or may simply be unable to do so at present. Using drugs is often a way of coping. Many people revert to using them once treatment is finished because they have not been helped to manage their lives without drugs. Learning to live without drugs is much harder than most people think, and may be tougher than overcoming physical addiction. The extra pressures of having a life-threatening illness make a wish to cling to the support drugs that seem to give all the more understandable.

Talking freely

You will need to be able to talk honestly. To do this you first need have a clear understanding of your own attitudes and of how you think and feel about a number of issues. You do not necessarily have to agree with the attitudes and ideas of the person you are caring for. You are both perfectly entitled to have your own opinions and beliefs. You should always feel free to say what you believe in a normal and straightforward way and should not need to compromise your own ideas or make excuses for them.

It is all too easy to assume that you know what the person you are caring for is feeling and thinking. It is far better to find out by asking. It is also vital not to trivialise or dismiss the answers you get. Whatever is said is probably important and so should be treated as such. It is also worth building a climate in which praise and encouragement are more common than criticism. This is often harder to do than it sounds, because many people find it easier to be negative than positive, and it can be harder to accept kind words than respond to harsh ones.

Think things through

Think things through very carefully before acting so that you don't have to change an impetuous decision. It is very easy to get drawn into any chaos and act impulsively. Try to step back and be objective. If you do make decisions which you have to change later you may appear to be fickle and inconsistent and make the person you are with feel insecure about the relationship and your intentions.

Working with others

Drug users have coped with HIV and AIDS in a number of ways. Some have turned to AIDS agencies for support, and have made full use of such services as the buddy network, mutual support groups and the range of practical help described in this book. Others have been helped by the hospital and community services, social workers, doctors and nurses. Some use drug organisations such as street agencies, needle exchanges or treatment centres. Some have formed their own self-help groups.

Details of the services and help offered by each of these organisations are given in this chapter and elsewhere in this book. You should fit in with whatever services are being used and try to find out about any others which may be useful. Without this support you are highly unlikely to be of use to the person you are caring for for any reasonable length of time. Many drug users have a wide variety of practical problems and may need considerable support in sorting them out. This can lead to confusion if there is no co-ordination between the services and help being received. It may be useful to try to work out some kind of care plan together.

Of course, some people who use drugs cope by themselves, isolated and unsupported. They may have had unfortunate experiences trying to get help in the past, they may have particular fears such as about having a child taken away, or more general suspicions of 'official' sources of help. If you are caring for someone who is receiving little or no help, you may find that you are called on to provide a great deal of emotional and practical support yourself. It may help to sound out some of the organisations, support groups or sources of information described in this book yourself. You could then go through the information you get with the person you are caring for to see if he or she would be willing to try any of them with your support.

Setting limits

Not surprisingly, drug users who are ill can experience intense feelings of depression, anger, frustration, loneliness, despair and distress. These emotions can appear in quick succession and without warning. They are less likely to have the support system that others may have to vent feelings and emotions. They may require more from you for this reason. Many carers find that they react by becoming upset themselves or begin to feel confused or helpless. Without good support, coping with this is difficult, and you can easily find yourself withdrawing from the situation. Conversely, it is also possible to become over-involved, so that you spend all your time and energy trying to help, and end up feeling tired and inadequate.

It is vital to set limits on what you plan to do. A basic ground rule for all carers is not to try to go beyond your own endurance. Decide what you can and can't do, do as much of this as you are able – and find someone else to do the rest, if you can. Equally, if you are asked to do something which you do not want to do, simply say no. If you attempt to do something you are reluctant to do this will probably be obvious to the person you are caring for, who may end up feeling guilty and rejected. You need also to be aware that it is quite possible to give too much help, which can mean that the person you are caring for becomes passive, dependent and helpless. Remember that the aim of enabling a person with AIDS to have as much control as possible over his or her life applies just as much to a drug user as it does to anyone else.

Common difficulties

Some areas have been problematical. Three are described below:

Talking about death

Many HIV-positive drug users go through a period during which they feel they have been given a death sentence. Some drug workers have not been trained to deal with feelings and fears about death, and disability; counselling in these may have to be arranged by you or even carried out by you. General information about counselling is on page 83.

Talking about sex

Sex for many people who use drugs is fraught with difficulties. Problems around having sex, sexuality and sexual identity can be common causes of relapses into some form of drug use. Drugs change the way people feel, think and behave, and information about safer sex is not always going to be put into practice by someone under the influence of drugs or alcohol. There are other complications, too. For example, some people who have been involved in prostitution may associate the use of condoms with their past and be reluctant to use them because of these associations. For someone who actively denies their illness, ignoring guidelines on safer sex can be a way of reinforcing a belief that nothing is wrong.

Even people who have stopped using drugs may have real feelings of uncertainty and anxiety about their ability to form relationships, which are further complicated by the questions of safer sex. Drug workers, drug users and carers may all have difficulty sometimes talking about sex frankly. This needs to be overcome.

Dealing with the attitudes of others

If you are caring for a drug user you can expect to meet many people who are unhelpful. Drug users with an HIV illness are rarely regarded just as people who are trying to cope with the possibly devastating consequences of the virus. They may be considered to be unworthy of care or help because they 'have just brought it on themselves'. Even now people talk readily about innocence and guilt in connection with AIDS. You have to be careful not to be affected by negative attitudes.

Taking care of yourself

The care that you give is going to be helpful only if you first learn how to take care of yourself. This is discussed fully on page 267, but has special significance for those who are caring for a drug user: he or she may lurch from problem to problem to such an extent that you may find you do not have time to consider yourself. If there is an existing support group locally, learn to use it. If not, consider starting one. Any local agency working in the field of drugs and HIV should be able to provide some resources ranging from arranging contact with other carers, providing rooms for meetings or becoming a point of contact.

Sources of help

At present very few services exist specifically to help drug users who have an HIV-related illness. Centres which aim to help people stop taking drugs do not usually have the facilities, staff or expertise to work with people who are ill. They are even less likely to be able to accommodate people who need terminal care. And organisations which do care for people who are terminally ill are sometimes unable to work with drug users, particularly those who are unable or unwilling to stop taking drugs. However, it is essential to get up-to-date information about what is available locally, as new services are being developed – see below.

Generally speaking, there are four different sources of help. These services themselves vary from area to area – information about how to find what is available in your area and elsewhere is given on page 239.

Drug advice, counselling and information agencies, often known as 'street agencies'

These are often run by voluntary organisations or Health Authorities. They vary in what they offer but you should generally expect a confidential, unbiased service which provides information, advice and various types of practical support. Particular services may include counselling, needle and syringe exchange (see page 238) or even child care facilities in some cases. Some agencies specialise in different fields: for example, some also advise on alcohol problems; some may specialise in helping specific groups such as young people.

Advisers have very specialised knowledge and have had experience of helping with all kinds of drug-related problems. They are likely to be the best initial source of advice for most people. All will discuss the options open to someone with an HIV-related illness, and will help anyone who is unsure of what to do or where to go next. They may also be able to help drug users deal with other problems, such as housing or money, either directly or by referring them on to a specialised service. Information is given to anyone who needs it – drug users, their families and friends. Street agencies are very easy to approach. If there is one locally, it is definitely worth finding out what it can provide.

National Health Service
GPs

GPs vary in their approach to drug users. Some are experienced and helpful. A good non-judgemental GP is an extremely useful ally and can help in various ways. Consulting a GP is usually the first step towards getting treatment or help. However, many GPs lack experience or willingness to work with drug users, and may not have the skills to do so effectively. Finding the right GP can be difficult. The person you are caring for may already know exactly which local doctors are knowledgeable and sympathetic. Otherwise, one of the local drug information agencies or AIDS Helpline may have information. Failing that, see page 49 for where to find general lists of local doctors. The GP can refer a drug user to an NHS hospital drug dependency unit (or centre or clinic). These don't exist in every District Health Authority so some travel may be involved.

Drug dependency units
(DDUs)

DDUs are usually based in hospitals, and can help drug users in a number of ways. Each DDU has its own policy – treatment may aim at helping people stop using drugs for a short while, or try to help them stabilise the amount they are taking, or aim at achieving total abstinence. Most treatment involves helping someone stop taking drugs by controlling withdrawal by the prescription of other drugs. This is not an easy process and can be physically and emotionally painful.

DDUs may treat people in the unit ('in-patient' treatment), or during regular visits ('out-patient' treatment). Some DDUs make home visits. Most staff have had training in HIV, and some provide considerable support and help for drug users with HIV.

In-patient treatment

This tends to last about six or seven weeks and it is usually possible for a determined person to stop taking drugs in this period, although staying off them when it is over can be difficult. Counselling, advice and continued support after treatment are therefore important, but the availability of these services varies from area to area. There may be a long waiting list for treatment due to a lack of beds, high demand and the large geographic areas most units have to cater for. Most treatment is in psychiatric or general wards which may not be suitable, particularly for people with HIV. In-patient treatment is usually reserved for people who are unable to stop using drugs while living at home.

Out-patient treatment

Most of the people treated by drug clinics are out-patients. Usually this means going to the clinic once a week or so for assessment and counselling. Drug users may be seen by a psychiatrist, nurse or social worker. They will usually be expected to have stopped using drugs after about six months, although some people need longer than this. Some clinics may have no special expertise in the special needs of people with an HIV illness, and many do not have any kind of visiting service for people who are too ill to attend the clinic regularly, so there may be practical difficulties.

If your health authority doesn't have a clinic, but does have some form of drug counselling service, treatment may be offered by a psychiatric unit in a hospital. In fact more drug users are referred to psychiatric hospitals and wards than to specialised drug clinics. Psychiatric facilities are rarely suitable for drug users and are even less suitable for a drug user with HIV, ARC or AIDS. If this is offered try to find out if there are any alternatives.

Community Drug Teams (CDTs)

All CDTs are linked to health authorities but they take a number of different forms. Some may be extensions of the DDU while others are independent. They offer help and support in a number of ways – liaising with GPs, providing advice, information, counselling and making home visits, for example.

Rehabilitation centres or therapeutic communities

People live in rehabilitation centres for anything from a couple of weeks to a year, learning to live without drugs in a controlled environment. Residents usually have to stop using drugs for at least 24 hours before being admitted. Individual centres differ in their approach to treatment; some have a very disciplined regime, others are more relaxed. Advice and information agencies should be able to give guidance on which sort of rehabilitation centre may be best for a particular individual. Most rehabilitation centres accept people from anywhere in the UK, but long waiting lists are common. Some centres now give priority to people with HIV-related illnesses.

Rehabilitation centres organised on the *Therapeutic Community* pattern require a relatively long stay and have a very structured programme, ending with gradual re-entry into the community. This treatment may last a year or more and involves giving up all drugs, although, at the latest stage, some alcohol may be allowed.

Some use what is known as the *Minnesota Method* which involves a shorter stay of about six weeks. Residents are encouraged to join in a programme of lectures, seminars, group and individual therapy as well as complete an extensive programme of reading and writing. The basic philosophy is that drug addiction *cannot* be cured but can be arrested as long as drugs which affect mood are *never* taken. Support in maintaining this total abstinence is given after the course of treatment by suggesting regular attendance at Narcotics Anonymous meetings – see below. Some people thought to be more in need are advised to spend the period following treatment (6–12 months) in a 'half-way house' where they will be in a protected environment. Nearly all clinics who offer the Minnesota Method are private. Some accept DSS payments but may expect residents to pay any amount outstanding in due course.

Drug-using people with AIDS have been divided in opinion about rehabilitation centres. Some found them to be helpful while others report distressing experiences because the centres were not able to meet their specific needs. Many centres use techniques based on confrontation and pressure, followed by attempts to 'rebuild' a person's sense of worth and self-esteem. Few aim to create a gentle, supportive environment where drug users can proceed at their own pace. It is difficult to say exactly what effect these methods, which can be long and painful, have on the health of people with AIDS. The fact that some treatments are phased over a comparatively long period also means that some people with HIV rule it out because they are not willing to commit themselves for so long.

Some centres now provide special facilities for people with an HIV-related illness and have also devised a more appropriate routine which, for example, allows more free time, accommodates special diets, and includes stress reduction exercises. There are a number of major issues to consider before starting a course of treatment at a rehabilitation centre.

Ceasing to take drugs

A 'drug-free' state may not be easy to maintain. Many people with HIV illnesses are prescribed pain-killing drugs, which may include opiates. These may be identical in many respects to the drugs the user is trying to avoid. This undermines the whole basis of treatment and can raise dilemmas for both staff and residents. People who have been prescribed opiates have found themselves unsupported and isolated in rehabilitation centres because they are considered to have reverted to using drugs.

Lack of medical facilities

Rehabilitation centres are not equipped to give medical care, and a person with AIDS who falls ill may find a programme of treatment is severely interrupted by spells in hospital. Most centres that admit people with HIV or AIDS will do so only on the condition that they will need no more nursing care than is already normally provided by the centre. This means that a drug user who is ill will have to wait for a period of remission before getting treatment. Most drug users, once they have decided they need treatment, tend to want it urgently, with as few delays as possible. They may not be prepared to wait until they have recovered from a bout of illness.

Inappropriate course of treatment

Some centres have rules which may be inappropriate for people who are ill. Some centres with a rigid discipline require residents to carry out domestic and other tasks at certain times, and demand that they attend certain group meetings. People with ARC or AIDS may often be too fatigued to comply. A rehabilitation centre can be lonely and frightening for a lone person with AIDS. Other drug users often feel uncomfortable in the presence of a drug user who has AIDS. It can raise issues that they don't want to think about, particularly if they have previously injected drugs and shared needles themselves. A person with AIDS can become an easy target for any bad feeling. This has caused some people to abandon treatment and return home unsupported. Often, they have had a feeling of having failed somehow, and so have ended up in a worse situation than they were in before.

For all these reasons it is essential that you make sure that the person you are caring for knows as much about any rehabilitation centre as possible. Talk to drug agencies nearest the centre and use local support groups to find anyone who has first-hand experience of it.

Two new residential units are being planned for 1991 which will cater for the special needs of people with HIV-related illnesses:

The *Turning Point* project, ROMA, is currently the only residential centre in the UK which accepts people who are currently notified drug dependents who are receiving treatment from a drug treatment centre or GP. Residents stay for up to six months, with an option for another six if it is agreed that this would be beneficial. Residents are encouraged to develop practical and personal skills and explore ways to reduce the use of drugs or become drug-free.

Turning Point are planning a new residential unit for drug users with AIDS; in the meantime a team of nurses at ROMA care for drug users with ARC or AIDS. It will be able to offer terminal care for people who are homeless or do not have other appropriate accommodation, and will provide short-term care for those who have periodic bouts of illness during which a high level of care is needed. People with AIDS will be able to stay for short periods to give their carers a break. [(See below for address)]

Phoenix House accepts people who have stopped using illegal drugs. A new residential unit – the Fountains Project is to be built in South-East London based on a therapeutic community (see above) but will be totally geared to the specific needs of people with HIV, ARC or AIDS. Eight of the 25 beds will be registered as nursing home beds so that full medical support, up to and including terminal care can be provided. If residents need specific hospital treatment during their stay, they will be able to return for follow-up care afterwards. Any drugs prescribed by a doctor for a medical condition will be accepted, including opiate-based analgesics. The building has been adapted for people with mobility problems. Phoenix House has over the years softened and changed the rigid regime of some therapeutic communities. Residents are allowed to have more say in their individual programme of treatment, which will take account of emotional, mental and physical health. It is a safe place where former drug users with HIV who are homeless or who live in unsuitable accommodation can get support.

They also help people living in the community and help in finding somewhere to live. People can refer themselves directly and do not need to go through a GP.

> Phoenix House
> 47–49 Borough High Street
> London SE1 1NB   01–407 2789

Phoenix House also have houses in Wirral, Sheffield, South Tyneside and in Forest Hill, London and are currently developing houses in Scotland and on the South-East coast. These do not have special nursing facilities, but people with HIV, ARC or AIDS will be able to use them.

City Roads (Crisis Intervention)

City Roads is a centre for people aged 16 or over who are in a drug-related crisis of any kind. It is the only such organisation in the UK. Referrals can be made by anyone, including the person in crisis. Following a referral the person in crisis is interviewed, usually within the day. Admissions are made strictly according to need but when City Roads can't admit someone they will help them find a centre which can. Residents have to stop taking drugs. If this is likely to cause health problems for people with HIV, City Roads will help them find a more suitable centre. Residents stay for about three weeks. They then either return to the community (City Roads will help arrange for support) or go on to another centre.

> City Roads (Crisis Intervention)
> 358 City Road
> London EC1V 2PY   01–278 8671 (24 hours)

Drug substitutes

People who have been taking heroin may be offered methadone as a substitute as part of a course of treatment. This can be prescribed by GPs (though some may be reluctant to do so) and drug treatment centres.

Methadone is a safer alternative to drugs sold on the street, which can be adulterated. Drug users often welcome the stability provided by a secure supply of methadone, which avoids the risks and effort involved in finding an illegal source. With a regular supply of methadone, some drug users can rebuild manageable and normal lives for themselves.

The only exceptional feature of this is that they continue to take an opiate-based drug. This may be as far as a drug user wants or is able to get towards total abstinence, and should not be undervalued.

Methadone is unlikely to be prescribed for lengthy periods, although there is mounting pressure to do this because of complications for people with AIDS if the supply is cut off and because it may reduce the incidence of sharing syringes. Even so, some clinics are likely to cut down the amount of drug they are prescribing. Even 'maintenance' prescriptions (giving a level dose of drug regularly) may be reduced in time. Methadone is most often used as a method of gradually weaning a user off all drugs. There is often a conflict of interest between what the clinic believes it should be doing, and what the drug user wants.

Methadone is unlikely to produce the sense of well-being or euphoria associated with heroin and other opiates. It just enables people to keep functioning and prevents withdrawal symptoms. For someone for whom getting intoxicated is a major part of their life, this is quite a sacrifice, and many drug users continue to use other drugs as well, although less frequently than before. If the clinic detects traces of these it may either cut down or cut off the supply of methadone. This may produce a crisis, and force a drug user back to using drugs as much as before. This can be dangerous because there is a possibility of overdose if someone starts again at a previous dosage level to which he or she is no longer tolerant. And the clinic may consider him or her to be unmotivated and unreliable and be unwilling to offer any more treatment.

Drug users who are ill may not always be fit enough to keep appointments at the clinic or collect prescriptions. The clinic needs to guarantee that treatment will be continued and prescriptions supplied if this happens. You may be able to help with arrangements, such as collecting prescriptions yourself (you will need authorisation), arranging for home visits or asking for drugs to be supplied to the hospital if the person you are caring for has been admitted.

Needle and syringe exchanges

Many people who became infected with HIV through sharing needles did so because they were unable to get clean equipment. Because of this needle exchange schemes have been set up in some areas. They may be run by voluntary organisations, drug dependency units or community drug teams. Additionally some pharmacists operate an exchange or sell needles and syringes to drug users.

Needle exchanges allow drug users to get a supply of clean equipment and dispose of used equipment easily and in absolute confidence. Even people who are HIV-positive should use clean needles because dirty needles can cause various health problems. A well-run local needle exchange may also be a source of information and support – they may be able to provide information on safer sex, condoms, arrange counselling and provide advice and practical help to drug users, their friends and families. To find out if there is a local needle exchange, contact SCODA (see page 241), any local drugs advice agency or the Health Education Unit (HEU) of your health authority, the National or a local AIDS helpline.

If there is no exchange, clean injecting equipment can sometimes be obtained from a local pharmacist. Pharmacists can supply equipment, at their own discretion, to drug users, although some are reluctant to do so. Some chemists may only be willing to sell to people who aren't drug users and may ask questions about whether you are a diabetic or not. Your local drugs agency or HEU may know which pharmacists provide this service. If you are already receiving help from the community nursing services you could ask them if they are willing to supply needles.

Disposal of used injection equipment should not be a problem even when there is no exchange to return it to. It can be safely disposed of inside a solid container such as a sealable tin, which the needle is unable to pierce, and put into the domestic waste. Alternatively, you can ask the community nursing services to provide a container called a *cin bin* and ask them to arrange for it to be collected. Do not overload the bin as it may burst and harm someone who handles it.

Self-help and community groups

Many drug users who become HIV-positive or cut down on their use of drugs lose their existing circle of friends – often the people they were using drugs with or getting drugs from. This can lead to feelings of isolation, which a carer, even if seen every day, can do little to alleviate. Drug users have no existing or identifiable community to turn to for support as gay men have had.

The most useful thing you may be able to do is to encourage a drug user to meet other people in a similar situation who are coping with many of the same problems. *Self-help groups* exist in most areas – sometimes they may be the only local service available. They provide help and advice to drug users, their families and friends. They may provide emotional support, practical help, and be a safe place to vent feelings at a pace a drug user feels comfortable with. They often take the form of discussion groups and some provide professional counsellors and telephone helplines. Self-help groups vary widely and have very different philosophies and styles. It is worth talking to them first to find out if they're appropriate to your needs.

Addresses

Groups set up to help drug users with HIV and AIDS
Mainliners

Mainliners is a charity set up to help and provide various services for drug users and former drug users affected by HIV and AIDS. They also provide advice and support for partners, families and people close to anyone with HIV and a history of drug use.

Mainliners is currently being relaunched. Contact them for details.

> Mainliners
> PO Box 125
> London SW9 8EF   01-274 4000 (x354)

Positively Women

Positively Women is a self-help group which started in London and is expanding its network through the UK. It works entirely with HIV-positive women, many of whom have been or are using drugs. They have an advice, counselling and information phone line.

Positively Women
333 Gray's Inn Road
London WC1X 8PX   01-837 9705

Specialist agencies

Information on drug agencies can be obtained from SCODA (see below) or The National AIDS Helpline (see page 56). You can hear a recorded list of phone contacts by dialling 100 and asking for Freefone Drug Problems, or by dialling 01-221 1175 direct. For lists of those in Scotland contact the Scottish Drugs Forum (see below). In Wales phone the All Wales Drugline (0222 383313) and in Northern Ireland phone the Northern Ireland Regional Drug Unit (0232 229808).

Institute for the Study of Drug Dependence

The ISDD is a research and information organisation with library. It publishes a wide range of pamphlets on a variety of drug issues.

ISDD
1–4 Hatton Place
Hatton Gardens
London EC1N 8ND   01-242 1878

Narcotics Anonymous

Narcotics Anonymous local groups are run and organised by addicts who have now stopped using drugs. They hold regular free meetings which have helped many people keep off drugs and develop their lives. Many people who went to their first meeting with no intention of giving up drugs completely have become regular attenders and have ceased to take drugs altogether. The aim of Narcotics Anonymous is to help people keep off drugs, and they do not offer help with HIV-related illnesses beyond this. They cannot provide the practical facilities such as medical care or treatment that people with an HIV-related illness may need. But, depending on the group, there may be mutual support from others also trying to come to terms with HIV, ARC or AIDS and a life without drugs. Some NA meetings are restricted to those who have a drug problem while others are open to families and friends as well. Details of local groups from:

Narcotics Anonymous
PO Box 417
London SW10 0DP   01-351 6794

National Association of Young People's Counselling and Advisory Services

NAYPCAS give information, by post only, on counselling and advisory services for young people throughout the country. They can provide a list of private counsellors who might be helpful when withdrawing from drugs.

NAYPCAS
17–23 Albion Street
Leicester LE1 6GD

RELEASE

RELEASE is an independent national agency concerned with the welfare of people using drugs. They have a confidential advice and information service on legal and drug-related problems, and a 24-hour emergency telephone service particularly for cases where someone has taken an overdose or been arrested.

RELEASE
169 Commercial Street
London E1 6BW   01-377 5905 (daytime); 01-603 8654 (24 hour helpline)

SCODA

SCODA (Standing Conference on Drug Abuse) is the umbrella organisation for work into drug misuse. They have information on all services available locally, covering all the types of help described in this chapter. With the BBC Drugwatch project they have compiled a directory of services, both local and national, in the UK. It costs £4 (including p+p) and is available from:

SCODA
1–4 Hatton Place
Hatton Gardens
London EC1V 8ND   01-430 2341

Scottish Drugs Forum

Information on organisations which offer help, support and advice in Scotland can be obtained from:

Scottish Drugs Forum
266 Clyde Street
Glasgow G1 4JH   041-221 1175

The South West Thames Regional Drug Dependence and Research Unit

The South West Thames Regional Drug Dependence and Research Unit has an advice line manned round the clock by professional staff. They will give advice and counselling by phone to drug users, families, friends, professional staff such as GPs and probation officers – and anyone else. They will have information about facilities and services in other areas.   Tel. 01-767 8711

TACADE

Education and training on drug-related subjects is given by TACADE (Teachers Advisory Council on Alcohol and Drug Education):

> TACADE
> 3rd Floor, Furness House
> Trafford Road
> Salford M5 2XJ   061-848 0351

Turning Point

Turning Point is the largest national voluntary organisation providing services for people with drug- and alcohol-related problems, their families and friends. They have a wide range of services to suit different individuals. These include residential rehabilitation, day-care programmes, information and support. Turning Point is extending its services for people with HIV and their carers. These include needle exchange, education, information and counselling.

> Turning Point
> CAP House
> 9–12 Long Lane
> London EC1A 9HA   01-606 3947

Groups for friends, family and carers

Although the organisations which specialise in giving help and advice about drugs will also help families and friends, there are several self-help groups specially for them.

ADFAM National

ADFAM National is an organisation for the families of drug users. It acts as a resource for the setting-up of self-help drug and family-centred projects such as helplines and befriending groups. HIV/AIDS awareness is included in their training. ADFAM also provides information, education and opportunities for discussion about drug use for families.

> ADFAM National
> 82 Old Brompton Road
> London SW7 3LQ   01-823 9313 (helpline)

Families Anonymous	Families Anonymous is an organisation of self-help groups for families and friends of those with a drug-related problem. There are 35 groups around the country – for details contact the head office.

> Families Anonymous
> 310 Finchley Road
> London NW3 7AG   01-731 8060 (24-hour answerphone)

OPUS	OPUS (Organisations for Parents Under Stress) have a counselling service and can supply information about various parents groups around the country.

> OPUS
> 106 Godstone Road
> Whyteleafe
> Surrey CR3 0EB   01-645 0505 (24-hour crisis line)

Samaritans	The Samaritans have a 24-hour telephone and face-to-face support service. They are listed under S in the phone book – see page 276 for more information.

Going private	There are private clinics which carry out all four of the types of service described above. Most charge fees, but some have assisted places which can be part-paid using Income Support payments. Some people have obtained grants towards the cost from health authorities, social services and charities. Private rehabilitation centres often use the Minnesota Model treatment described above, and rely on persuading the user to take responsibility for his or her own life and recovery. Most private clinics will suggest that their clients continue treatment by attending groups run by Narcotics Anonymous. A high success rate is claimed, and the treatment has the advantage of being manageably short (six or seven weeks, usually). For those who can afford it, this may be an option worth considering if suitable treatment under the NHS cannot be obtained.

Drug laws	The Misuse of Drugs Act is intended to prevent the non-medical use of certain drugs. Drugs controlled under the Act are placed in different classes, depending on how harmful the drug is thought to be and on the penalties associated with offences involving that drug.

Class A drugs have the highest penalties – up to life imprisonment for production or trafficking and up to seven years for illegal possession. Heroin, opium, LSD and cocaine are in this class.

Class B drugs include cannabis, amphetamines and some sedatives, and have lower penalties (up to five years for possession). Any Class B drug which is prepared or used for injection automatically becomes a Class A drug.

Class C drugs incur the lowest penalties and include tranquillisers and some sedatives – penalties can include up to two years for illegal possession.

15 *Haemophilia*

Most of the information in this book will apply to the needs of people with haemophilia who are HIV-positive or who have ARC or AIDS. However, there are some differences.

Support

Although the agencies set up to help AIDS will help anyone, some people with haemophilia may not feel them to be appropriate if they seem to focus on the needs of gay men. The Haemophilia Society has a long-established system of local support groups, and many of these offer considerable support to people with an HIV infection, as well as to those who are ill and their carers.

Health

Some people with haemophilia have developed great strength and resilience in meeting its challenge and this is an enormous advantage in fighting HIV. They are used to regular hospital visits and are generally very aware of their own health. Another advantage is that hospitals will have a detailed record of their medical history, which can make monitoring health and the state of the immune system easier. As haemophilia is itself a potentially life-threatening condition, they may even regard HIV as just another complication and cope with it extremely well.

Nursing

Some older people with haemophilia may be used to frequent bouts of being confined to bed. An additional problem posed by HIV is that resting in bed may aggravate problems with joints. People with haemophilia can also be prone to more bleeding episodes due to HIV complications and experience fatigue.

Financial problems

Before treatment with Factor VIII became available in the late seventies, haemophilia often severely restricted schooling and the ability to work. As a consequence many older people with haemophilia have had severe financial problems, sometimes compounded because haemophilia is hereditary and can therefore affect more than one member of the family. Chapter 9 describes the various welfare and private benefits available, including funds provided by the government for people with haemophilia.

Emotional aspects

Haemophilia is passed from mothers (who are carriers, but not usually affected) to their sons. There is a 50/50 chance that the daughters of carrier mothers will be carriers themselves. All daughters of men with haemophilia are carriers. This can lead to sadness which can affect the relationships between the male and female sides of the family. Those infected with HIV may have very strong feelings of anger and resentment about this double burden. Parents who have in the past unknowingly given children infected blood products (before heat-treated factor VIII and blood screening) may also have additional feelings of guilt about this. Another problem may be that more than one family member is infected with HIV. Working your way through this minefield may be difficult – see page 203 for sources of help.

Information

If you have been caring for someone with haemophilia for some time you will already be familiar with the condition. If not, contact:

The Haemophilia Society
123 Westminster Bridge Road
London SE1 7HR   01-928 2020

Alternatively, get in touch with a Haemophilia Centre (there are around 110 of these up and down the country). Many larger centres have social workers who are able to help families and their carers, and liaise with outside agencies. Some provide all primary care, so some people with haemophilia may have very little contact with a GP.

16

When someone dies

Various practical arrangements have to be made following a death. Sometimes it can be helpful to be absorbed in these at a time of loss. Although the arrangements described below sound quite complicated what happens is usually quite straight-forward. The professional people you will come across are usually able to guide you through in a supportive and understanding way.

If a death occurs the first thing you should do is tell the doctor. When a death has been expected the doctor may not consider it necessary to come round, or may not do so immediately. You need to tell the doctor if the body is going to be cremated, as he or she then has to examine it, and arrange for another doctor to do so, too. The doctor will issue a medical certificate of the cause of death – this is legally necessary so that the death can be registered.

When someone dies in hospital the medical certificate of the cause of death is usually completed by a hospital doctor. The death certificate is a legal document and doctors have to put down the real cause of death. However, this may be the opportunistic infection which caused it, and the certificate need not mention AIDS. If you are concerned about what the certificate may say, talk to the doctor.

A death has to be reported by a doctor to a coroner if the doctor did not attend the person at all during the last illness. If the doctor was treating the patient but had not seen him or her within the last 14 days (28 days in Northern Ireland), nor viewed the body, the death will also have to be reported to the coroner. Other circumstances in which a death must be reported to a coroner include cases of suicide, deaths which occurred in suspicious circumstances, death which occurred within 24 hours of being admitted to a casualty department, and those which took place during a surgical operation or before recovery from the effects of an anaesthetic.

If the coroner decides that the death must be investigated further, a post-mortem may be required, in which case the death cannot be registered until the coroner provides a certficate. An interim certificate can be issued, which is usually enough for starting to deal with the estate. If there is to be a post-mortem without an inquest the registrar will issue the appropriate death certificate – currently £2.

In Scotland if a medical certificate of the cause of death cannot be given, the facts must be reported to the procurator fiscal. The procurator fiscal, amongst other responsibilities, carries out similar duties to coroners in England and Wales.

When a death occurs at home, you can ask a funeral director to come and take the body away or it can be laid out at home. This involves washing the body, stopping up natural orifices with cotton wool and a napkin, dressing and tidying. When someone has died of an infection, a funeral director may wear protective clothing. Although this is done as discreetly as possible it may be upsetting. When someone dies in hospital you have to arrange with the funeral director for the body to be taken away from the hospital mortuary. A relative or executor will have to sign a form authorising the funeral director to do this. If the body is to be cremated, the necessary forms will be completed at the hospital – see below.

Hospitals often want to carry out a post-mortem examination to find out more about the cause of death. They cannot do so without permission from the next of kin. Whoever goes to the hospital following a death should be prepared to say whether the next of kin will allow the hospital to carry out the post-mortem, and if so, to sign a consent form.

Registering a death

The doctor will write out a medical certificate of the cause of death. The doctor may give this to you to take to the registrar covering the area where the death took place (or, in Scotland, it may also be taken to the office for the district where the dead person normally lived, provided this is in Scotland), or may send it directly. The death has to be registered within five days (eight days in Scotland). In England and Wales you are allowed another nine days after the first five if the registrar has been given written confirmation that the medical certificate of the cause of death has been signed by a doctor. A list of the local registrars of births and deaths can usually be found in doctors' surgeries, post offices, public libraries and other public buildings. You do not usually need an appointment.

The law allows only certain people to provide information to the registrar. These can be relatives who live or happen to be in the sub-district of the registrar or a relative who was present during the death or during the last illness If there is no eligible relative the informant can be anyone who was present at the death, someone living in the house who knew of the death or the person responsible for making the funeral arrangements. (In Scotland any relative of the person who has died, any person present at the death, the person's executor or other legal representative, the occupier of the premises where the death took place, or any other person who has knowledge of the particulars, can be the informant.)

The registrar will ask you for details of the date of death, where it occurred, the sex, names and surname of the dead person, including maiden name, where appropriate. Also needed will be the person's date and place of birth, occupation and last address. (In Scotland the registrar will need to know in addition the time of death, and details of spouses and parents.) The registrar will ask for the person's medical card. If you don't have it you will be given a pre-paid envelope to send it later. Once a death has been registered, the registrar issues a green certificate, known as the disposal certificate. (Coroners give an order for burial or certificate for cremation.) Neither burial nor cremation can take place without this. In Scotland there is no disposal certificate: the registrar will give you a certificate of registration of death which is used instead.

After registration

Certified copies of the entry of death in the register are known as 'death certificates'. You will need them when arranging the affairs of the person who has died. You will need different versions of the death certificate for other purposes such as obtaining probate, claiming life insurance or national insurance or social security benefits. All are obtained from the registrar, who will advise you about the different certificates you will need.

Repatriation

If the person who has died is to be flown elsewhere for burial, there are various organisations who can undertake this. Some specialise in HIV-related deaths. Contact the National Association of Funeral Directors (NAFD) for details (address on page 250), or an AIDS helpline.

The funeral

If the person who has died has left no specific instructions, the decision about whether to cremate or bury is usually made by the next of kin or executor. The wishes of the dead person are usually followed, although there is no legal obligation to do so. Nearly all funerals are arranged and carried out by undertakers, now called 'funeral directors'. They co-ordinate all arrangements, from the laying out of the body (which they call 'first offices') through to burial or cremation. They also will make sure you have completed all the necessary documents, and will pay the various fees which arise (to cemetery or cremation authority, clergy and so on). These charges are added to the final bill. Members of the trade association – the National Association of Funeral Directors (NAFD) – undertake to follow a code of practice. This means that they should always give you full information about services and prices, provide a written estimate of all charges and a detailed breakdown of all costs afterwards. They all offer a simple or 'basic' funeral, if required. In this case a breakdown will not be given of how the total charge will be made up. The lowest price of a simple funeral is unlikely to be less than £350. Members of the NAFD treat someone who has died from an HIV-related death in the same way as anyone else.

You can – and should – ask funeral directors to quote for a funeral. If you intend to spend no more than a limited sum, tell the funeral director so and do not be persuaded into anything you do not really want. You can have preliminary discussions over the telephone, but arrangements are concluded face to face. The funeral director should provide a price list for the different types of funeral offered. Ask for some time to consider these and discuss them with other people concerned. You will need to think about what extras you may need in the way of transport, flowers, notices, catering and so on. Try to keep track of how much each of these extras will cost before you commit yourself. Funeral directors will understand if payment cannot be made until the estate is settled. Pre-payment schemes make it possible for a person to pay for a funeral in advance, in instalments. The National Association of Funeral Directors operate a scheme through their members.

National Association of Funeral Directors
618 Warwick Road
Solihull
West Midlands
B91 1AA   021-711 1343

Some co-operative societies also have a pre-payment scheme. With some, every time a payment is paid, a voucher for half of this amount will be given to the payer. This voucher can be spent in the co-operative society's stores on anything other than food. If you are interested in this, check with your local co-operative society to find out if a pre-payment scheme exists in your area.

Some local authorities provide a municipal funeral service, and others are looking into the possibility of doing so. These are likely to be cheaper than any other alternatives – arrangements would be made with local funeral directors to provide a simple, low-cost service for local residents. Contact your local authority.

If no one is able to pay for the funeral, your local authority may arrange and pay for it if necessary. In these circumstances you must get in touch with the local authority social services or environmental health department before trying to make any arrangements yourself; costs cannot be refunded afterwards. If you do arrange for a funeral, but cannot afford to pay for it, you may be able to claim some of the cost from the Social Fund – see page 170.

You can arrange for the body to be left at home until the funeral, if you wish. Most people arrange for it to go to the undertakers. Usually relatives and (with their permission) friends can go and see the body there; sometimes it is necessary to make an appointment. Embalming or 'preservative' or 'hygienic' treatment (which is not the same as the ancient Egyptian process of mummification) is used to preserve the body for a temporary period. Undertakers will not usually embalm anyone who has died from an HIV-related illness because it involves replacing blood with a solution of formalin and other chemicals. This means that burial or cremation may have to take place within three or four days of the death.

Ceremonies

Most religious denominations have some form of funeral ceremony. They can usually be adapted to suit those concerned. If you are arranging for the funeral of someone of a particular faith you should contact the equivalent of the local parish priest to find out what has to be done. Your funeral director may be able to help.

There is no need to have a religious ceremony, or indeed any kind of ceremony, at a funeral. However, because such ceremonies are usual, it is necessary to make it clear early on that no service will be needed. A non-religious ceremony can take any form, provided it is decent and orderly. If you need it, you can get help and advice from the following organisations:

British Humanist Association
13 Prince of Wales Terrace
London W8 5PG   01-937 2341

The BHA give guidelines for a non-religious funeral in *Humanist Funeral Ceremonies* – £3 including p+p.

The National Secular Society
702 Holloway Road
London N18 3NL   01-272 1266

The Rationalist Press Association
88 Islington High Street
London N1 8EW   01-226 7251

The South Place Ethical Society
Conway Hall
25 Red Lion Square
London WC1R 4RL   01-242 8032

Burial in a churchyard

Some people have a right by law or custom to be buried in a parish churchyard – ex-parishioners and non-parishioners with family graves or whose close relatives have been buried there and those who die within the parish. Other people whose permanent address is within the parish, whether Christian or not, are also, in theory, entitled to be buried in the parish churchyard. In practice, there may be no space. It is up to the vicar, rector or priest in charge to decide if anyone outside these groups can be buried in the churchyard, and on the fee to charge. Most kirkyards in Scotland are administered by the social work department of the local authority; a grave is referred to as a lair.

Burial in a cemetery

Most cemeteries are non-denominational and are run by either a local authority or a private company. Some are owned by particular denominations and can be used only by members of that faith. Some cemeteries have ground dedicated to or reserved for people of a specific religious faith and a separate section of general ground.

Cremation

No one can be cremated until the cause of death has been established, although preliminary arrangements for the cremation service can be made as soon as the death has occurred. Cremation cannot normally be applied for until after the death has been registered and the registrar's certificate issued or a coroner's certificate given.

Three forms usually have to be filled in – one by the next of kin and the others by three doctors. Forms can be obtained from the crematorium and usually from a funeral director. Form A is the application for cremation, and has to be filled in by the executor, or next of kin, and countersigned by a householder who knows the person signing. Form B has to be completed by the doctor who attended the person who died during the last illness. The doctor has to see the body before completing the form. Form C has to be completed by another doctor, who also has to see the body. When someone dies in hospital, the hospital will fill in these forms. The final authority to cremate is given on form F and is signed by a doctor who is the crematorium's medical referee. He or she usually does this on the basis of the medical evidence on forms A, B and C and the registrar's certificate.

Forms B and C are not needed when a coroner has issued a certificate for cremation. When a death is reported to a coroner, you must tell the coroner (or the funeral director who will instruct the coroner) from the outset that you want the body to be cremated. If you don't you will have to go back to get another certificate.

Most crematoria are run by local authorities. They have non-denominational chapels, but it is usually up to you or the funeral director to make arrangements for the service, if any. If you do have a religious service, it will have to be fairly short, unless a special booking is made for a longer period. If you want to take away the cremated remains, you can collect them 24 hours after the cremation, in a container provided by the funeral director or crematorium. Alternatively, the crematorium will post them. The funeral director may be willing to collect the remains for you.

After the funeral

None of the property of the person who has died should be given away or sold until probate (if there is a will) or letters of administration (if there isn't) have been granted. The person's representative must inform the bank (who will stop payment of all cheques and banker's orders); notify any other institution where the person had an account (any savings will be temporarily frozen) and notify the tax inspector. After the grant of probate or letters of administration the representative will settle debts, obtain payment of any life insurance policy, and transfer the ownership of any house, shares or other property.

In Scotland dealing with someone's estate is quite different. Before the estate can be administered the sheriff usually has to confirm the authority of the executor named in the will (or the one appointed by the court if there was no will). The forms required for getting this confirmation can be obtained from the commissionary department of the local sheriff court or from:

The Capital Taxes Office
16 Picardy Place
Edinburgh EH1 2NB   031-556 8511

Confirmation forms ask the executor to give an 'inventory' of all property, cash, personal effects, furniture, car and so on. A solicitor can help with this if necessary and the sheriff court may also give help, especially with small estates worth under £17,000. The Capital Taxes Office will tell you if any inheritance tax is due, and how much it comes to. Completed forms are lodged at the sheriff court in the area where the deceased lived. Confirmation is returned by post. This has to be shown to anyone with an interest in the estate. Confirmation is not always required – for example if property is held in common by the person who has died and another by title which contains a 'survivorship destination' so that it passes to the survivor.

For further brief information about wills see page 104. ALBA at the Scottish AIDS Monitor (see page 58) has legal advisors who can help.

For more information, see *What to Do When Someone Dies*, from which most of this chapter was drawn. Consumers' Association also publishes an Action Pack, *How to Sort Out Someone's Will* (which covers England and Wales) see page 290.

17

Bereavement

Most people get very little preparation for dealing with death. Children are not taught about death in a way which would make coping with it any easier. Adults may rarely discuss it, and so act in an unsure and clumsy way when faced with a dying or grieving person. The taboos which prevent death being treated in a commonplace way continue to make it difficult for dying people to die peacefully. Grieving itself may be made harder by a world which is embarrassed by any obvious sign of distress and keeps its distance from it. Any open display of anguish following a death is often discouraged, despite the fact that everyone who has loved or is loved will experience bereavement at some time in their lives.

Caring for someone who is dying will be one of the most difficult experiences anyone has to face. Not only will there be profound emotions, but there will be a host of practical details to be dealt with. Various alterations in one's life, both will have to be faced at a time when one feels least able to deal with them.

Caring for someone with AIDS brings additional problems. Some carers will also be HIV-positive, and the possibility of developing ARC or AIDS themselves will be a nagging and fundamental concern, sometimes causing acute fear and anxiety. An increasing number of people will have known more than one person who has died from an HIV-related illness. A series of losses can be almost unbearable.

Finally, there may be less support and sympathy for carers of people with AIDS. You may meet prejudice even at this most difficult time. Families may stay aloof from gay partners and deny them the support of sharing grief. Sometimes the support services and facilities are so firmly geared to the loss of heterosexual partners that they will be irrelevant. Some families and some carers may feel that it is necessary to be secretive about the illness, so carers are more isolated than if they were caring for someone with a more socially acceptable condition.

Grieving

Grieving is a natural and important process. We need to grieve. It allows us to mark and appreciate our relationship with the person we mourn, yet many people hide their grief, and sometimes don't even acknowledge it fully to themselves. Not being able to show grief can result in distressing feelings of varying kinds later on. And the stress caused by unexpressed sorrow can actually be dangerous for people who are HIV-positive.

Many people just feel numb after being told of the diagnosis. This is a natural way of coping with the situation – you shouldn't worry that your lack of apparent feeling means that you don't care or that something is wrong with you. Another common experience is profound fear. Among partners there are often very specific fears, notably worries about being able to go it alone after a partner's death, worries about money or accommodation and a fear of having or developing AIDS him or herself. Alternatively, fear may not be of anything in particular but a general apprehension about the future.

It is easy for resentment to build up, sometimes even unconsciously. Some people feel guilt or anger when a person close to them is dying, but never really come to recognise or admit the reasons for these feelings. They may be due, for example, to resentment that opportunities for a continuing and developing relationship have been cut short, or guilt at remaining well while a partner is ill. Discussing any such feelings may help. The more you can express yourself early on, the less difficulty you may have later. It is easy to feel guilt about going out or remaining involved in things other than the illness of the person you are caring for at such a time. However, you should not exclude all other activities. You may find that you need a break from the situation from time to time, and need to make sure that you will be be fresh and strong enough for the times when you really are needed.

Caring for someone who is dying

Elisabeth Kubler-Ross, an American doctor who has worked extensively with people who are terminally ill, has described different stages they may face in her book *On Death and Dying*. These include:

Denial

Denial is very common at the time of diagnosis, but usually fades. People may be open about their illness to some, while denying it to others. Some may switch from denial to a perfectly realistic appraisal of the situation within short periods. Let the person with AIDS decide how much reality is to be faced at a time.

Anger

Anger, rage and resentment are all common reactions. 'Why me?' 'What have I done to deserve this?' These can be especially distressing not only because of their force and vehemence but because the anger may be directed at you. It is important not to take this personally. You may be the target of the anger but are not the real cause of it. Sometimes anger will be expressed by making unreasonable demands. This may be a way of reminding you that the person you are looking after is still alive, and the demands will probably lessen as you demonstrate your love and understanding.

Depression

Depression about the impending loss of life is difficult to deal with. You may find a 'looking on the bright side' Pollyanna type of attitude may help you, but this may not be helpful to the person you are caring for. Kubler-Ross believes that you should not make it hard for anyone to contemplate their own death, nor should you feel you have to tell somebody who is dying not to be sad. Often this stage may be silent – you may communicate just by the touch of a hand.

Acceptance

Once anxieties and anguish have been worked through, it is possible to reach acceptance and peace.

'If a patient has had enough time (i.e. is not faced with sudden imminent death) and has been given some help in working through the previously described stages, he will reach a stage during which he is neither depressed nor angry about his "fate". He will have been able to express his previous feelings, his envy for the living and the healthy, his anger at those who do not have to face their end so soon. He will have mourned the impending loss of so many meaningful people and places and he will contemplate his coming end with a certain degree of quiet expectation. He will be tired and, in most cases, quite weak. He will also have a need to doze off or to sleep often and in brief intervals, which is different from the need to sleep during the times of depression. This is not a sleep of avoidance or a period of rest to get relief from pain, discomfort, or itching. It is a gradually increasing need to extend the hours of sleep very similar to that of the newborn child but in reverse order. It is not a resigned and hopeless "giving up", a sense of "what's the use?" or "I just cannot fight it any longer", though we hear such statements too. (They also indicate the beginning of the end of the struggle, but the latter are not indications of acceptance.)' from *On Death and Dying* by kind permission of the publishers.

You should allow the person you are looking after to express their feelings to you. They may rage, cry or just want to give voice to their fears and fantasies. They will be unable to do this unless you take the time just to sit quietly and listen. Kubler-Ross observes that it is this which makes a gradual and peaceful separation possible. She goes on to point out that acceptance is not a happy stage, but one in which the person is really void of all feeling; the struggle is over. At this time they may want to be left, and not concerned with the outside world. Visits may be better kept short, and the number of visitors kept to those the person with AIDS really wants to see. At this time your task, if you are the main carer, may be just to provide continuity and reassurance. Not much may be said and perhaps you will communicate only by touch, but your presence will be important.

Of course, everybody is different, and some or all of the stages described above may not appear or they may appear in a different order. However, they do suggest the kinds of feelings and moods you may meet. Your guideline should be to let the person take charge, and to listen. He or she will raise any issues felt to be important without any prompting. But you have to provide the atmosphere in which this is possible. An important part of your role is to let the person express and come to terms with his or her own feelings.

If you hope that an awkward subject will not be mentioned, the person will probably sense your attitude and be unable to talk about it. This is particularly true about dying itself, where it is sometimes the carer rather than the dying person who is unable to face up to things. When the person wants to talk about death, you should make it possible for this to happen easily. He or she may make an oblique reference to it just to test the water, and will continue only if you seem to be open about it. The worst thing you can do is pretend. Apart from anything else there is no time for 'deception games' of this kind, however strongly you feel they may help. Dying people are often able to face their situation in a refreshingly honest way, any attempts by you to disguise the truth will be unhelpful.

You may find that there are a number of loose ends the person you are caring for wants to tidy up. These may be practical arrangements, business affairs or relationships. You should listen and follow these leads without trying to take over. Your job is to help with tasks the person can no longer manage and give support when needed. Find out what is wanted and do whatever is necessary.

Towards the end some friends may continue to visit after the time when the person feels that loose ends have been tied up and that particular relationship has been 'completed': 'I can't keep on saying goodbye'. Your job will be to explain gently to the visitor that the time has come for a final farewell.

> *Dying people become like gurus. There is a mad rush of people trying to cope with the feelings that come up for them. A dying person doesn't want to cope with everyone else's garbage . . . it's OK to release his garbage but not vice versa*

Some people wish to talk about someone else who has died, perhaps because of misunderstandings which were never resolved or regrets about past events which can now no longer be put right. Again, your role as carer is really to listen and prompt only when it seems necessary. For example, it may help to ask what the person would have liked to have said, and talk through the situation from there.

One mother described how she and her son talked a lot on the night he died. He said 'the only reason I'm fighting this is because I'll miss you'. The mother felt he was asking for her permission to die.

After someone has died

> *Helped a lot to see him, very peaceful, after he'd died. I didn't plan to go, I just decided I wanted to go, I drove, I can't remember getting there. It helped*

Losing anyone you love is one of the most agonising experiences you may have to face. The realisation that someone who has been around, who has shared so much, is no longer there is difficult to come to terms with. For some time afterwards you may continue to see the person – in shops, on buses. You may think you hear his or her voice. You may wake up in the middle of the night to the stark realisation that it wasn't all a dream after all. All these are symptoms of shock, and they may be very slow to disappear. Some people have great difficulty in accepting that someone who was close to them has really died.

People who have been through a bereavement have said that they felt numb just after their loved one died. All feeling seemed to disappear as if they were under an anaesthetic. You may feel a great distance between yourself and other people and the world in general. At this stage it is often possible to cope with immediate practical tasks with some degree of coolness. This is the moment, too, when you, who have been providing support for someone who was dying, no longer need to do so. Instead, it has become you who needs support, and you should not hesitate to turn to friends and family for their help.

The funeral brings home the finality of the loss, and it is after this that many people become aware of a deep and aching void. You may have a desperate need to have someone to talk to; perhaps someone who also knew the person who has died who can share some of your thoughts, appreciation and memories. Sometimes it can be hard to find anyone like this to confide in. Many people don't realise that the shock and realisation of a bereavement really begins to tell some time after the funeral, and they may not be aware of your need to talk. Most people are uncomfortable talking about death and feel uneasy or inadequate when they are with someone who is showing signs of grief.

These signs – crying, trembling, hysteria or whatever – are a way of releasing feelings naturally and should be welcomed. Many people who offer to help try to stop you feeling grief because they may think it's embarrassing, or a sign of weakness. Ignore them. Sharp emotional pain, sobbing, gusts of anger are all common experiences. You may find you have sudden outbursts of any of these. Whatever you feel, express it. Talk, cry or scream if you need to. Grief should not be hurried. Just follow you own feelings and do whatever you find gives you the most comfort. Your feelings may be a way of searching for the person who has died, or may express anxiety, insecurity or just plain anger. If you are lucky you will have friends who will understand and help you through. In time you can expect to reach a stage where you can accept all that has happened.

You may have to rethink the way you organise your life to adjust to a new routine. The lack of someone to discuss things with may be the time when you become most aware of the gap in your life. It may help to try face these practical difficulties one by one, without letting yourself be defeated by thoughts of how much there is to do and the difficulty of it all. Worst of all there is no one there at times when you need someone. Advice and help offered by friends and relatives may be no substitute and you may even feel that they are an intrusion. Sometimes it is difficult to share your feelings with the family, particularly if the person who has died was gay and they have rejected or have expressed uneasiness about your relationship with him.

Nevertheless, if you have a network of friends or relatives to whom you are close during this difficult period, they will probably be the best support in the end. If you are not so fortunate, or if you wish to get some outside help, various organisations (and some individuals) offer bereavement counselling – they will talk and guide you through this difficult period, help you express your own feelings and work your way through all the various emotions you will be feeling. Counselling may be given individually or take place in a group. Being with other people who are in the same situation, sharing your common feelings and concerns, may be a great source of strength and comfort. To find out what exists in your area contact your local AIDS helpline, or one of the organisations below.

CRUSE

CRUSE is a national organisation originally set up to offer help and support for widows and their children. They now help with bereavement whatever your relationship with the person who has died. They have over 150 local branches throughout the country. A local branch or the national headquarters will be able to tell you about your nearest source of help. CRUSE have their own counselling services, too. All the branch counsellors are volunteers, so it is worth asking if a particular counsellor has any experience of bereavement associated with AIDS. Counselling may be given individually or in groups.

> CRUSE
> Cruse House, 126 Sheen Road
> Richmond
> Surrey TW9 1UR   01-940 4818

Compassionate Friends

The Compassionate Friends is a nationwide organisation which aims to help parents whose child has died (at any age and of any cause) by putting them in touch with other parents who have lost a son or daughter. They support the newly bereaved through telephone calls, letters and personal visits. Regional branches hold regular meetings.

> Compassionate Friends
> 6 Denmark Street
> Bristol BS1 5DQ   (0272) 292778

London Lighthouse	London Lighthouse run a bereavement counselling course and also have plans for a bereavement support group. For more information, contact the Counselling and Training Department on 01-792 1200.
Terrence Higgins Trust	The Starting Over group provide support for people who have lost a partner as a result of an HIV-related illness, and helps them find ways to make a new start. Meetings are held weekly at the THT. They are mainly attended by partners (men and women) although friends and family are also welcome. Group members can also contact each other outside of these meetings for mutual support. See also page 203 for details of other support groups and page 57 for information about the THT.
Gay Bereavement Project	Telephone counselling can be remarkably comforting. The Gay Bereavement Project is a charity which will give support and counselling by telephone. They were originally set up to help the surviving partner of a gay relationship and that remains their main aim, but in an emergency they would try to help parents, brothers and sisters or friends. They are particularly aware of the problems of not being able to grieve openly and the difficulties of finding someone to talk to who fully understands the situation. They also give advice about making wills – see page 105.

Gay Bereavement Project
Unitarian Rooms
Hoop Lane
London NW11   01-455 8894. Their helpline operates from 7pm to 12pm, 7 days a week. See chapter 4 for more information about counselling.

18 Religious and spiritual support

Some people with HIV have felt that the infection (or even being gay), has cut them off from the support and understanding of their church. Sometimes this has been because they have felt guilty about their lifestyle or actions. Others have been put off approaching a church or other religious institution because of reports of religious intolerance in the press, or because of a longstanding fear that the church would not be sympathetic or understanding.

Various religious-based groups have now been set up to meet the needs of people with HIV. Most offer counselling and the opportunity to discuss things from a religious perspective. Some may offer healing services, advice on bereavement or funerals or whatever spiritual support is needed. Some organise and provide practical support of a non-judgemental and non-evangelising nature. New groups are being set up, so for more recent information check with your AIDS helpline, or the Terrence Higgins Trust Interfaith group, which brings together people from many religious groups to provide understanding and support. They or the groups described below should also be able to put you in touch with sympathetic clerics.

Interfaith group
Terrence Higgins Trust
52–54 Gray's Inn Road
London WC1X 8JU   01-831 0330

Manchester Interfaith Group

The Interfaith group in Manchester give advice and information to people living in the North-West. They offer practical help with religious activities and provide spiritual support. They can give information about other sources of religious help in the North-West.

> Interfaith group
> St Peter's House
> Precinct Centre
> Oxford Road
> Manchester M13 9GH   061-273 1465

Inter-denominational
Christian groups
ACET

ACET (AIDS, care, education and training) is a Christian-based organisation with mainly Christian staff. Their prime aim is to provide practical support and education – see page 65.

> ACET
> PO Box 1323
> London W5 5TF   01-840 7879

CARA

CARA (Care and Resources for People Affected by AIDS/HIV) is an umbrella organisation for groups that give support – both pastoral and religious – to people with HIV and their families. They train volunteers, organise retreats and run an HIV/ARC and AIDS support group in London. So far other groups exist in Birmingham, London and Sussex. CARA can also supply details of any similar groups in your area.

> CARA
> The Basement, 178 Lancaster Road
> London W11 1QU   01-792 8299

Christian Action on AIDS

Christian Action on AIDS works mainly to inform religious groups about AIDS but is affiliated with a number of groups around the country which organise retreats and offer counselling from a Christian point of view. If there isn't a group near you they will try to find another organisation which may be able to help.

> Christian Action on AIDS
> PO Box 76
> Hereford HR1 1JX   (0432) 268167

Lesbian and Gay Christian Movement

The Lesbian and Gay Christian Movement have counsellors available to talk about any problems and can advise on sympathetic clergy. Send an SAE for an information pack.

BM 6914
London WC1N 3XX   01-587 1235

Reaching Out

Reaching Out is a Christian-based listening centre open to anyone.

Reaching Out
Flat 3b Langham Mansions
Earl's Court Square
London SW5 9UP   01-373 1330

Welsh clergy

If you live in Wales and would like a list of members of the clergy who offer AIDS counselling, contact the address below, stating your denomination:

Social Care Resource Centre
University of Wales College of Cardiff
37 Corbett Road
Cardiff CF1 3EB   (0222) 874000 (x5386)

Anglican churches

To find out about associated caring schemes or support groups, contact:

General Synod of the Church of England
Board for Social Responsibility
Church House, Great Smith Street
London SW1P 3NZ   01-222 9011

Buddhism

The Buddhist Hospice Trust is a small charity which gives spiritual counselling from a Buddhist perspective for people who are terminally ill or bereaved. They have set up a support network in London – the Ananda Network – and hope to establish similar groups around the country.

Buddhist Hospice Trust
PO Box 51
Herne Bay CT6 6TP

Ananda Network
5 Grayswood Point
Norley Vale
London SW15 4BT   01-789 6170

Catholic church
Catholic AIDS Link

Catholic AIDS Link (CAL) are a national support network of Catholics caring voluntarily or professionally for people with HIV or AIDS. Some of their volunteers have HIV themselves. They give support to Catholics affected by HIV in any way. This may include referral to other support groups. They have regular services and occasional international gatherings where carers can exchange experiences. Small emergency grants are sometimes available.

CAL
PO Box 646
London E9 6QP   01-986 0807

Jewish faith
The Jewish AIDS Trust

The Jewish AIDS Trust offers counselling to people with AIDS, their families, carers and friends – face to face if you live in London, otherwise by phone or letter. Leave a message on their answerphone and someone will ring you back. They also organise educational talks and workshops.

Jewish AIDS Trust
PO Box 799
London N3 3PN   01-455 6449

Jewish Lesbian and Gay Helpline

The Jewish Lesbian and Gay Helpline is a nationwide information and counselling service. They have information about social groups, events, religious services and have a list of helpful rabbis. Counselling is given on religious and other issues, including HIV. Tel. 01-706 3123 (Monday and Thursday evenings, 7pm to 10pm)

Others

The Metropolitan Community Church is a Christian Ecumenical Church with groups around the country – phone for details. They offer counselling services either at their offices or in your home.

Metropolitan Community Church
2a Sistoria Road
London SW12 9QT   01-675 6761

19 Caring for the carer

It is important that you, as a carer, should remain as fit as possible and accept that taking care of yourself is an important part of your task.

> *The majority of carers are very poor at looking after themselves. They can flatten their batteries and start having a negative effect on the people they are trying to help*

Much of this chapter is for people who are caring fairly intensively for someone who needs quite a lot of support. It is worth restating that this does not happen to everybody and many people with AIDS do not need or want help to this extent. Even those that do may need it only for short periods.

Ways of making caring easier

Sharing tasks with others

One of the biggest differences between carers who have experienced great stress and those who have coped well was in the support the *carer* received from friends and professionals. Without this the isolation can become very destructive:

I am given very little gratitude for all I do for him. We are together 24 hours a day . . . I would like more people to visit him to let me go out more

Some carers don't want other people involved. This may be because they want to show their love by caring alone and may not want anyone else breaking into a private situation. All too often carers wish to be 'strong' and to be everything and do everything themselves. Although they may do this in the utmost good faith the result may be a poor quality of care. Think carefully if this applies to you. Are you sure that such an attitude isn't just possessiveness? And are you sure that you can really cope alone? By contrast, some carers become angry because they feel that they are being unfairly imposed on, and that others aren't doing their bit.

Many friends and relatives will be willing to help, although you may have to take the initiative and ask them. This is sometimes difficult to do, but you may find that the people you approach just didn't know how or what to offer. Asking for help doesn't mean you can't cope but is a sign you are trying to do so in the most efficient way. It is important to ask for help as you need it; otherwise you may find more and more tasks are falling to you by default.

Later in this chapter we summarise where in this book you can find information about the professional help you can get for common practical problems.

Get support for yourself

Support can make a tremendous difference. Sometimes carers question their right to ask for support for themselves. But it is likely that there will come a time when you will need someone to talk to, to sort out a particular problem, or hold on to:

I regret not getting help not so much because of the benefit I would have got, but more because of the help I might have been able to give to my lover. Looking back I feel I should have gone out and looked for help but at the time I was just overwhelmed by the situation

If you don't feel well supported consider what steps you can take to get help. Bear in mind that you may need much more support in the future. If you get to know the people involved before there are any major problems you will have a network to call on and will be more prepared if a crisis does occur.

Share your feelings

Caring for and being cared for are really interdependent: the more one is cared for the easier it is to care for others. However difficult or traumatic the task, you will be able to handle it more easily if there are other people you can talk to. Frustrations which are bottled up can fester and cause all sorts of problems later.

Talking over problems and sharing your worries is one of the most useful things you can do. Just the act of putting your emotions or fears into words may help. Often the role of a confidant is to allow someone to talk and get rid of their worries rather than coming up with solutions. Whom you talk to is up to you. You may want to talk to different people about different things. People you know well may be easier to confide in, although it is sometimes more productive to talk to someone who does not know you or the person you are caring for. You may get a new perspective from someone outside the situation. Some people prefer to talk to a counsellor, or to one of the professional people involved with the person with AIDS. The test is to find someone with whom you feel sympathy. Information about counsellors and counselling is in chapter 4.

Meeting other carers

It is easy to feel that no one understands. But many carers have found when they have discussed things that they have shared similar experiences – even feelings they have felt guilty about such as wishing it was all over, or feelings of anger or resentment. Even if you usually prefer not to talk about your feelings it may help to try. It is much easier – and often a relief – to talk when other people are describing experiences which reflect your own.

I find the support group that I'm in of tremendous help. But there is a low uptake of these resources because of the lack of awareness that the carers also have to be cared for, and carers don't think about their own needs

I need some form of supportive group to relieve the pressure on my friends . . . possibly a situation where another couple in the same situation could be found to share their experiences and problems

See page 277 for the support groups for carers which have so far been set up. It is essential to check with your local AIDS helpline, or with the National AIDS Helpline, to get details of the latest developments.

Drawing on the support of family and friends

Most of all I would have liked somebody to talk to in the last few months of the person's illness, especially as I'd had to move house to a bungalow so that I could cope with the wheelchair etc. and found it so much of a responsibility.

Friends and family can be a major positive source of practical and emotional support. They may be particularly important outside larger cities, where professional and voluntary help can be hard to find. But it is often up to you to make it clear that you welcome company or need practical help – people often need to be sure they are welcome, and that their friendship and help is appreciated.

Sometimes there are difficulties. AIDS is an emotive word and may frighten some people away. Although it is impossible to generalise, negative reactions of this kind can be fairly short-lived, at least among close relatives and friends. You may need to be patient and let any initial shock and fear fade naturally rather than risk permanent damage by being aggressive. Unfortunately, it is not always easy to be patient when you may feel vulnerable yourself. It will help a great deal to discuss such problems with others who have dealt with difficult families, and had to cope with rejection. Some information about family therapy is given on page 90.

Avoiding 'tunnelling'

Avoid living in a tunnel of HIV. Keep up your other interests, remain in contact with friends and try to go out. Nobody expects you to be on call 24 hours a day. Keeping in touch with friends can be distracting and is time-consuming. It often becomes easier not to bother. But you can become isolated if you give undivided attention to the person you are caring for. And it is difficult not to become stale or even obsessed unless you can step back from the situation from time to time. A woebegone carer will do no good to anybody, least of all to anyone who is ill. This doesn't mean adopting an air of false jollity or an artificial mask of any kind. But you may need to give yourself permission to feel happy at times, and not feel guilty about keeping your other interests afloat. Remember that a positive attitude and cheerfulness are infectious!

Dealing with exhaustion

It is easy to become overworked and overtired. You may also feel that nothing can be done about it and become depressed. A starting point is to review what you are doing to see if there are any tasks which needn't be done, or done so well or so often. Secondly, be sure that you have enlisted all the help you can from friends, family and professionals. You may be able to find more time to sleep by rearranging your day. If you are having problems sleeping, see page 273.

Coping with strong feelings

Depression, anger, resentment and guilt are all strong feelings and can be extremely destructive. They can all result in your becoming ill, mentally and physically.

Try to find a way of relaxing – see page 272.
Try to get a break – see page 280.

If you feel angry, it often helps to find your own safety valve – taking time alone, for example, venting anger by punching pillows or whatever. It is important to find someone you can talk to, confide in, or even shout at, if necessary. If you find it easier, talk to a counsellor. Your GP may also be able to advise.

Stress

Stress can have many causes. You may have very basic fears about the future, about your job, or about your relationship. Watching someone develop the symptoms of an extremely debilitating illness is tormenting. Yet you have to summon up the energy to cope with the everyday tasks of caring, sometimes with little obvious encouragement. You may have an underlying feeling that all your efforts are futile, and that you are getting nowhere. And there are added burdens if it is necessary to be secretive about the nature of the illness. It is not surprising that many carers become very depressed themselves.

I cry a lot now and get panicky about the future. I feel I'm under more stress because I'm more scared about what is going to happen

It would be a rare person indeed who did not experience stress in this situation. You may feel that you can handle only a certain number of problems, uncertainties or changes at any one time and there may be times when all the different pressures on you seem intolerable. If stress cannot be avoided, ways have to be found to keep it under control and cope with it.

Symptoms of stress

Stress can have physical and mental symptoms – or both. Physical symptoms have been mistaken for signs of other illnesses, including HIV infection, because they can be so similar. They include chest pains, diarrhoea, headaches, nausea, breathing difficulties, twitches and, at times of acute emotional stress, even fainting. Some illnesses are thought to be related to stress and others may be complicated or worsened by it. It is thought by some that stress may depress the body's immune system. Stress control for people who are themselves HIV-positive is therefore particularly important.

Anxiety and depression are the two emotional conditions most often associated with stress. Someone who is anxious is likely to be extremely tense and jumpy and is likely to over-react. Quite trivial events can turn into a major crisis. Hope and despair can be experienced in turn, often in quick succession. Physical symptoms such as sweating, tightness in the chest, a sinking feeling in the stomach and increased pulse rate may appear as well. Severe anxiety can bring on a persistent sense of dread and foreboding. It becomes difficult to pay attention and simple tasks become hard to carry out. Many people who suffer from anxiety have *panic attacks*. These are acute periods of extreme anxiety which often seem to come on for no apparent reason, perhaps in the street, out shopping or on public transport. Besides strong fear, physical symptoms may include your heart pumping furiously, sweating, difficulty in breathing, nausea and trembling. You may feel sick or think you are about to faint or otherwise make a fool of yourself. It is easy to persuade yourself that you are ill.

Depression is a long-lasting mood of bleakness and pessimism to which there seems no end. Most carers are likely to experience depression at some time – many people feel an underlying sadness much of the time. However, a depression which darkens your whole life and excludes all else, which is not even pierced by temporary moments of relief or humour, is an illness. People with depressive illness lose interest in activities, reject their friends and generally begin not to care about anything. Guilt and a feeling of being unworthy or inferior are also common. Physical symptoms may include headaches, backache, insomnia, loss of appetite and constipation.

Dealing with stress

- Give yourself *permission* to relax. It is easy to feel that it is your tension which holds you together, and therefore you need to preserve it. Some people cope by being 'busy' and concentrate on activities which take their mind off things.
- Remind yourself about the good things in your life. List those that help make you feel relaxed, such as sleeping, reading or having a bath. Allow yourself more time to do these things. Take time off.
- Be aware of your thoughts. Are you blaming yourself or feeling guilty about

anything? Do you feel hopeless about the future and feel agitated a lot of the time? Are you much more irritable or absent-minded than usual? These are all quite common and normal feelings. They are all signs that you may need to talk things over with a friend or counsellor. Consider ways of relaxing – some are described below.

Alexander technique

If you have muscular tension and aches, and are having difficulty physically relaxing, the Alexander technique may help. It involves relearning how to use muscles and avoid tension by improving your balance, movement and posture. Learning how to adopt better physical posture often helps you to unwind mentally, too, and encourages good breathing and the ability to relax parts of the body. However, it may take a fair number of lessons to make a noticeable improvement. For a list of teachers, send an SAE to:

The Society of Teachers of the Alexander Technique
10 London House
266 Fulham Road
London SW10 9EL   01-351 0828

Massage

Massage can help you relax, as well as reduce muscular tension and the pain it causes. It can also be very comforting because the physical contact involved can make you feel cared for. Some physiotherapists or occupational therapists attached to GP clinics will demonstrate how to carry out simple massage.

Complementary therapies

Diagnosis and treatment used in complementary medicine concentrate on finding and correcting the ways in which the body is out of tune. You may find the idea and practice of alternative therapies attractive and appealing. See page 200 for details of where to find more information and how to find a good practitioner.

Sleeping

Problems with sleeping are very common indeed – difficulty in getting to sleep, waking in the night, waking too early and sleeping intermittently or too shallowly. People under stress often find they can't stop thinking about their problems at night, and toss and turn. Sleep, when it does come, is often filled with disturbing dreams. Waking up in a sweat and panic is common. Sleeping pills will not deal with the cause of insomnia, so consider talking about your situation with someone. You may find it easier to get to sleep if you can get into a routine. Try to get to bed at the same time every night, and get up at the same time. Exercise, reading or relaxing in some way before you go to bed may help. A warm bath and warm drink (not coffee or tea, which are stimulants) may also help. Some relaxation techniques – making up stories, adding and multiplication games or repetitive exercises like counting sheep – may do the trick. Or you could try relaxing muscles in each part of your body in turn.

Exercise

Exercise may help relieve stress. It may be particularly beneficial to get involved with sports and pastimes in which others are involved – even regular walks with friends. You can also exercise at home – *Keeping Fit While Caring* by Christine Darby (Family Welfare Association, £2.95) shows you how to move, lift and bath someone who can't do these tasks alone and includes some keep-fit exercises. *Physical Fitness* by the Royal Canadian Air Force (Penguin Books, £1.99) gives details of short daily keep-fit routines for men and women.

Physical relaxation techniques

Physical relaxation can help ease fatigue and help you cope with stress. It is often seen as a preventive therapy which can also help to boost your own healing system. One common method of physical relaxation is to concentrate on different parts of the body and relax those muscles in turn. Your local library or education authority will tell you if there are any evening classes in relaxation. The charity *Relaxation for Living* will send you a list of local classes, and they also run a correspondence course for people who cannot attend classes. They also publish leaflets and tapes for relaxation (for adults and children), insomnia and nervous illness. Send a large SAE for details.

> Relaxation for Living
> 29 Burwood Park Road
> Walton-on-Thames
> Surrey KT12 5LH   (0932) 227826

Tapes and books which help with stress are also produced by Lifeskills.

> Lifeskills
> 3 Brighton Road
> London N2 8JU   01-346 9646

Immunity (see page 107) has two relaxation tapes (£5.50 each including postage.)

Overcoming positive HIV-test stress and handling anxiety
Tranquillisers

People under stress sometimes take minor tranquillisers (sedatives) such as Valium, Librium or Ativan during the day, and Mogadon at night. These have a calming effect, and may make problems seem less insistent in the short term. While they may make the immediate situation easier to deal with, they only mask the stress. You will still have to deal with the cause later. The side effects of minor tranquillisers can include drowsiness, dulled sensitivity and, after a time, lessened intellectual capabilities. Minor tranquillisers are effective only for a few weeks if used continuously. Both minor tranquillisers and sleeping pills of the benzodiazepine group can cause dependence. If you take them for two weeks or more you may have unpleasant withdrawal symptoms when you try to stop. Depression can often be helped by talking, or a change in attitude or lifestyle. If you have reached the point where life seems unbearable or your body seems to be quite unlike its usual self, you may benefit from anti-depressants. These can be prescribed by your GP. They take 10 to 14 days to have any affect; and this is followed up by another course of treatment which usually lasts from six to eight weeks. People who are prescribed anti-depressants must be careful about taking other drugs and alcohol. Before you consider taking any drugs to help with anxiety or depression discuss your situation fully with your GP. Many will be able to help you deal with anxiety without using drugs but by counselling.

MIND

MIND (National Association for Mental Health) produce special reports on anti-depressants, minor tranquillisers and other drugs used to treat mental health problems. These cost 25p each. Information and help can be obtained from the MIND head office or from the regional offices or local MIND groups.

> MIND
> 22 Harley Street
> London W1N 2ED   01-637 0741

TRANX

TRANX give information, advice and counselling to people who want to overcome an addiction to minor tranquillisers and sleeping pills. They publish a quarterly newsletter, and sell a tape (£6.50) which gives advice and takes you through a course of relaxation.

> TRANX (UK) Ltd (National Tranquilliser Advice Centre)
> 25a Masons Avenue
> Wealdstone
> Harrow HA3 5AH   01-427 2065; 01-427 2827 (24-hour answering)

Help for people who feel stress

The Fellowship of Depressives Anonymous

The Fellowship of Depressives Anonymous (FDA) brings depressives together for mutual support. Open meetings are also held bi-monthly in different places; anyone interested in the work of the FDA can attend. Send an SAE to:

Fellowship of Depressives Anonymous
36 Chestnut Avenue
Beverley
North Humberside HU17 9QU   (0482) 860619

Depressives Associated

Depressives Associated is a self-help organisation with support groups throughout Britain. They also provide information to people who suffer from depression and to their relatives or friends who want to help. Send an SAE (9 × 6 in) to:

Depressives Associated
PO Box 5
Castle Town
Portland
Dorset DT5 1BQ

The Samaritans

The Samaritans is a charity that provides emotional support around the clock for those for whom life may be getting too much to bear. Confidential help is offered by telephone, face-to-face and by letter. There are more than 180 branches throughout the UK and the Republic of Ireland.

Healthline

Healthline is a library of taped messages, written by medical experts, which you can listen to over the phone. Each tape will tell you about a particular subject including stress, acute anxiety and depression, and where to go for more information. Dial 01-980 4848 between 2pm and 10pm on any day, including weekends. The operator will play the tape you choose. For a list of all the tapes you can listen to write to Box 499, London E2 9PU. Healthline is free (apart from the cost of the telephone call) and confidential – the operator will not ask for your name or for any other information. (Healthline should not be confused with Healthcall, which is similar but the call is charged at a much higher rate.)

Support for carers

HIV groups

The Terrence Higgins Trust (THT) provides various forms of support for carers. Get in touch with the Trust to find out if any others have been set up recently. The National AIDS Helpline will tell you what's available locally.

The Family Support Network (FSN)

The Network will provide support and counselling for anyone related to or closely involved with someone who has ARC, AIDS or who is HIV-positive. Regular meetings are held at the THT and in West London; other meetings may be set up elsewhere in the future. These provide an opportunity to share feelings, talk about problems and draw on the advice, help and fellow feeling offered by people who have had similar experiences. Group members offer each other mutual support and friendship outside the meetings, too. If you don't want or are not ready to attend a group there is also an extensive home visiting service in London. Visits are made at the time of an initial crisis, when things have settled down after this, and when extra help is needed. Visits are sometimes spread over a year or more, so you can expect long-term support.

For people outside London support can be given by telephone. You need to make an appointment so that you can talk for as long as is necessary – an hour is about average. The Network also counsels people after a bereavement. All the Network's counsellors have been trained either as family counsellors or by the THT, or both. All conversations and meetings are completely confidential.

The Family Support Network also has a hospitality service. Relatives or friends who come to London to visit a person with HIV can be given up to five days' bed and breakfast accommodation in a volunteer's home. This may be enough to cover the visit or at least will give you enough time to find cheap accommodation – the Network may be able to help you with this, too. The Network is also developing resources to give families in crisis a break. Accommodation is given to families (not to people with AIDS themselves) for periods of up to five days.

Other initiatives being considered include a support group for children with HIV-positive parents. It would help children cope with such things as problems connected with sexuality, bereavement and the difficulties of having to keep things secret from friends and schoolmates. Services are continually expanding – check with the Network for the latest information. Contact the Network through THT or THT's helpline. There is also a 24-hour telephone line on 01-436 6253.

Lovers' Support Group

The anxieties and concerns felt by partners can be immense. They are also very personal and may be difficult to talk about or even express in words. The Lovers' Support Group provides an opportunity for people in similar situations to meet and share their feelings and concerns. It is often easier to talk to people who may be sharing the same feelings as yourself. It is also often a relief to be able to talk freely particularly if you have to be careful about what you say at other times – at work, for instance, or even when with the person you are caring for.

Meetings are held weekly at the THT and are mainly attended by partners although friends and family are also welcome. Groups are very informal and what is discussed largely depends on what happens to emerge at a particular meeting. Group members are, of course, free to contact each other outside of these meetings for mutual support. Contact the THT (see page 57) for more information. See also page 262 for details of the Starting Over group, which will give help following a bereavement.

SAM

Family support is also given by the Scottish AIDS Monitor (SAM) – contact the counselling and training officer at the Edinburgh and Glasgow office – address on page 58. 'Friends' is a support group for carers – friends, lovers or relatives – of someone who has an HIV-related illness based in Edinburgh, and for those who have been bereaved. Counsellors are trained and group therapy sessions are held every two weeks. Contact the Scottish AIDS Monitor (see page 58) for details.

CASTLE

Caring and Sharing Together in Lothian and Edinburgh (CASTLE) is also based in Edinburgh and is for families, friends and relatives of people with HIV or AIDS. Meetings are held fortnightly and ten sessions make up a programme. For more information, contact:

Social Work Department
Bangour General Hospital
West Lothian EH52 6LR   (0506) 811334

Body Positive

Body Positive was set up as a self-help group for people who are HIV-positive. It has extended its help and counselling services, including training weekends, to anyone who is concerned with HIV-related issues. See also page 59.

The Lantern Trust

The Lantern Trust has been set up to provide training courses for professional people who care for people with HIV. It has a resource pack which contains leaflets on drug use, housing, psychological matters, employment, HIV and children and nursing. More titles are planned. These leaflets have been produced for organisations to distribute themselves. However, they are also free to individuals who send an SAE to:

The Lantern Trust
72 Honey Lane
Waltham Abbey
Essex EN9 3BS   (0992) 714900

General support for carers

It is likely that your local area will have some form of support scheme for carers generally. At the very least there are likely to be regular meetings where carers can meet each other and discuss common concerns. Carers' groups are an immense source of mutual support and information. Acting as a group you will also have a stronger voice if you want to press for new services, more resources or information. If there is no group specifically for carers of people with AIDS, a group for carers generally may exist. Your local social services department should have details, particularly as many are organised from there.

You may feel that a general group of carers may not be appropriate for you, or you may find that an existing group is not really tackling the issues that you face. If you feel that such a group is important, and would like to start one, explore the idea with your local AIDS organisation and the social services department. *Caring Together* by Judy Wilson (from the National Extension College, 18 Brooklands Avenue, Cambridge CB2 2HN, price £3.95) aims to help carers start and run their own group. It has been written for carers generally, not specifically for the carers of people with AIDS.

The Carers' National Association

This organisation aims to bring carers together in local groups, give information about local services and welfare rights for carers, and they sometimes provide respite care. They provide an opportunity for carers to come together, share experiences and provide support for each other. Most of their members will be caring for an elderly relative or a disabled spouse. While all should be able to help with local information some may not be particularly attuned to the needs of carers of people with AIDS, and may not be the best source of emotional support.

Contact the Carers' National Association headquarters for information about your nearest group. They will be able to tell you if it has been involved with any other carers of people with AIDS.

Carers' National Association
29 Chilworth Mews
London W2 3RG   01-724 7776

Taking time off

It is important to take time off. You may need time to sort out the practical side of your own life, or simply need a break. You may even just want time to rest or sleep. Many people feel guilty about taking time away from the person they are caring for, particularly when they are giving a great deal of time and help. However, taking time off may make it possible for you to continue to care and show that you care. People who haven't taken breaks sometimes get to the stage where they can no longer cope with the effort and stress, and end up treating the person they're caring for in a hostile way. Sometimes a crisis completely unconnected with caring for someone means you have to take time off. It is a good idea to consider beforehand what you will do in such circumstances, so that you will not be caught unprepared.

Taking a Break is a guide published by the Kings Fund Informal Caring Programme. The booklet is free, and gives full details of how you can arrange to get a break. Single free copies are available from Taking a Break, Newcastle upon Tyne NE85 2AQ. It lists four symptoms, any one of which may be a sign that you need a break:

- frequently losing your temper
- sleeping badly, for no obvious reason
- feeling tired all the time
- finding that even small things which once didn't bother you are getting on top of you.

We are grateful for permission to publish the following edited extracts which describe some of the pressures carers are under when trying to consider a break.

'Most carers, even those taking breaks, are unsure about whether having a break is the right thing to do. You may want a break yet feel guilty for wanting to get away, even for a short time. You may believe that you should be able to cope and that to let someone else take over is an admission of failure. Sometimes it can seem that a relief carer copes better than you do, and this can make you feel inadequate. You may think your family should help more, or find it difficult to turn down family help if it doesn't work out.

'Many carers don't like to make a fuss, or believe that others are worse off than they are, and so tell themselves that they don't need a break.

'It is also not unusual for carers to become frustrated and angry because breaks are difficult to arrange, too infrequent, or unsuitable. You may feel that the professionals who should assist you are unconcerned and unhelpful. Some carers feel that they have to "fight" for everything including services that the person they look after is entitled to. Many just don't have the energy to take on the additional work of arranging a break on top of what can be the day-to-day exhaustion of caring.

'You may tell yourself that you can't take a break because the person you look after won't like it and will refuse to co-operate. Indeed, it is not unusual for people to resist the idea of being looked after by someone else. This can exert a lot of pressure on you, which may leave you feeling resentful toward the person you look after and very indecisive about having a break.

'It's probably true that most carers worry about the effect a break will have on the person they look after. But you are likely to be most anxious the first time, especially if they are going away from home. You may worry in case the person is unhappy without you and that they will be homesick. And, of course, you will be concerned in case others are not able to look after them as well as you do. You may fear their particular needs will not be seen to. You may be worried in case the break makes the person's condition worse.

'All these worries and anxieties are normal, and are often justified. There is no simple solution. You will want to take the feelings of the person you are caring for into account, and the strength of his or her feelings. Try to resolve any difficulties by talking about them. An honest talk should stop the person with AIDS interpreting your need for a break as a kind of desertion or as a sign that you care less, or that your strength of feeling or support is fading: explain that you need a break from the work, not the person'.

You then need to consider the options.

'Respite care' is the name often given to schemes which allow carers to take time off. You may come across other labels too – relief care, short-term care, phased care and social admission are examples. In various forms it is provided by social service departments, health authorities, voluntary organisations and even private individuals. Sometimes these agencies may organise facilities in cooperation with each other. What's on offer will vary considerably from area to area and generally local services are not sufficient to meet the need for them. Some services are free and others are not. Some support groups have introduced sitting services and the two London AIDS hospices have facilities for respite care. Details are given below.

To find out what is available in your area try your local AIDS helpline or ask any of the professional staff you are in contact with – social worker, doctor, health visitor or whomever. Otherwise contact your social services department or health authority direct. The national addresses of the main voluntary organisations concerned are given in Chapter 3. To find local private organisations which provide the services described below, look under 'nursing' in the Yellow Pages.

Like most local services, most respite care services not provided by specialist organisations have not been set up to care for people with AIDS, and it is essential to check the agency first. In particular talk to the individual concerned to make sure that he or she has a positive and realistic attitude. An unsympathetic or ignorant carer would be counter-productive.

Care at home

Arranging for relief care at home causes the least disruption, and one-to-one care provides the most continuity. However, the demand for these services is great, and it may be difficult to arrange for help at short notice.

Sitting services

Social services departments, voluntary organisations, district health authorities and some private agencies may have 'sitting' services. These may be known by other names such as 'family support' or 'bridge-in' schemes. Sitters, usually volunteers who have had personal experience of caring, normally stay for a few hours, day or evening, although some stay overnight. They may not be able to offer any nursing care or do more than keep company or help in simple ways. Apart from private agencies which charge, services may be free or there may be only a small fee. Some schemes are aimed at particular groups of people (the elderly, for example), and your situation may not fit their rules. AIDS organisations which at the time of writing run sitting services are ACET (page 65) and London Lighthouse (page 67).

'Care attendant' schemes

Several voluntary organisations now provide trained staff ('care attendants') who provide relief care for periods ranging from a few hours to a few days, although they will not usually stay overnight. The aim is to relieve you of work and worry for a short period. To do this they will try to fit in with your routine so that the person you are looking after has minimal disruption to face. Care attendants are trained and can cope with most tasks, but they are not meant to take over from services provided by other people such as district nurses or home helps. Social services departments and health authorities sometimes offer similar services. Demand for care attendants is heavy, so there may be a waiting list. Schemes may also be known as Family Support Services, or Extended Home Help Schemes. They are often free but sometimes a small charge is made. Private agencies also have care attendant schemes; rates vary.

Crossroads

The Association of Crossroads Care Attendant Schemes have about 140 separate schemes in England, Scotland, Wales and Northern Ireland. Crossroads Scotland Care Attendant Schemes have 46 schemes in Scotland. Each is autonomous and makes its own decisions about priorities and the type of service it offers. They are independent of health authorities and social services departments but work in cooperation with them.

The majority of Crossroads schemes aim to help people with a mental or physical handicap. Because of this people with AIDS may not qualify for help, but it is worth contacting your local scheme – some do offer care to anybody who needs it, resources permitting. And it is certainly reasonable to say that a person handicapped by AIDS is no less needy than someone affected for some other reason. Nearly all Crossroads schemes make no charge, although donations are welcome. Your social services department will know of Crossroads schemes in your area, or you can contact:

> Association of Crossroads Care Attendant Schemes
> 10 Regent Place
> Rugby
> Warwickshire CV21 2PN   (0788) 73653

or, in Scotland:

> Crossroads Scotland Care Attendant Schemes
> 24 George Square
> Glasgow G2 1EG   041-226 3793

Nursing services

If cancer is involved you may be able to arrange for a Marie Curie nurse to stay overnight or for part of the day – see page 52.

Live-in help

Private agencies and voluntary organisations (including a few care attendant schemes) can provide live-in help while you go away. Some organisations use volunteers, others have trained staff or qualified nurses. Some health authorities supply district nurses for short periods, but most do not. Charges made by private agencies vary and these can be expensive.

You can, of course, employ someone yourself to help. The most difficult part of this arrangement can be finding the right person. You will have to do this through contacts, advertising (perhaps in an AIDS newsletter) or by asking a local support organisation to help. You will need to interview any applicants – with other people if possible, as it is invaluable to have a second (or even third) opinion.

When choosing someone, it may be more important to find someone with the right attitudes and approach than someone with, say, the best nursing qualifications. Organising a trial period is a useful way of making sure the arrangement will work before finally committing yourself.

You, as the employer, will be responsible for deducting your employee's National Insurance Contributions if he or she earns £43 or more a week. You then have to pay this plus your own NI contribution (as the employer) to the Inland Revenue, together with any PAYE income tax deductions (this will depend on the employee's personal tax allowance). Your tax office (under Inland Revenue in the phone book) will help you organise this. You may be able to get financial help towards the cost of hiring a helper from the DSS (see page 155).

Some tips from *Taking a Break*: Prepare for the break by involving the person you care for in planning the break, and talking about the reasons for it, and how it may do you both good. An experienced 'outside' person, such as a social worker or nurse, may help you both see things more clearly and ease any tensions.

Introduce the new carer gradually. At the beginning it helps if you are both there. You may have some teething problems and you may feel that having a relief carer is creating more work for you. However, the carer should be able to take over more of these tasks as he or she becomes more familiar with the situation. Give the carer all the information you can – about the particular needs of the person you are caring for, details of any medication, diet, likes and dislikes, habits and routines. It may be useful to demonstrate how you carry out certain tasks. Tell any other helpers, such as the district nurse and home help, when the relief carer will be there.

Care away from home

Respite care, for periods of a few days up to several weeks, is offered by some hospices – see page 69. It may be possible to arrange for a temporary stay in a hospital, either in a ward or a special unit in a NHS hospital – contact your doctor. This is free, but may affect social security benefits – see Chapter 9.

Day hospitals

Day hospitals run by the health authority are centres for people who are ill, disabled or elderly who live at home but require medical treatment, specialised care or rehabilitation. They are staffed by health and welfare workers and provide care and opportunities for carers to have a break. They vary from area to area: some may only be for people with specific illnesses; some may only open at certain times; some may offer occupational therapy or recreational facilities. They are all part of the NHS and so are free, as is transport by ambulance there and back. Day hospital care has to be organised through a GP.

At present there are no day hospitals provided by the NHS specifically for people with AIDS. Some health authorities may be considering this or may be able to give information about whether existing centres are appropriate.

The Kobler Centre in Fulham has an out-patients' clinic for people with AIDS, and also medical day care facilities. The London Lighthouse and Sussex AIDS Day Centre in Brighton are also places where people with AIDS can spend part of the day – these are described on page 67. Mildmay Mission (see page 72) is also planning a day centre.

Breaks in a residential home

Residential homes run by the social services, and by voluntary and private organisations, which take people for a short stay to give their carers a break. They are, however, usually for older people, or for those with specific disabilities, and may not be appropriate for this and other reasons. There are agencies such as Carematch (01-609 9966) will give advice on choosing a home, or you can check with your social services department.

Marie Curie Cancer Care

The Marie Curie Cancer Care organisations has eleven residential homes for people with cancer. Between them they have 400 beds. They all offer short-term admissions to provide relatives with a rest period. You can apply to any home, irrespective of where you live – contact the matron first. Priority is based on medical and social need, but not all homes have waiting lists. Information and addresses from:

Marie Curie Cancer Care
28 Belgrave Square
London SW1X 8QG   01-235 3325

21 Rutland Street
Edinburgh EH1 2AH   031-229 8332

Holidays

Another way of organising a break is to go on holiday together. This may not be a solution if you need a rest from the whole situation, but may be a welcome and invigorating change of routine if you want to introduce some variety or forget about domestic chores for a time. See page 176 for information about charities which may help you out with financial difficulties. If special care is needed, you will have to think about choosing a holiday to fit in with these needs.

The Holiday Care Service

The Holiday Care Service has information on hotels, self-catering apartments, package holidays and holiday facilities for people with special needs. This includes accommodation which is accessible for wheelchair users, and also accommodation where extra care is provided. They provide information only; you have to make travel and booking arrangements yourself.

To date, the Holiday Care Service has not so far undertaken any specific research regarding facilities for people who have AIDS. The service does not usually communicate direct with providers of accommodation about individual clients. It is up to those going on holiday to discuss any special needs with them direct, and to make a judgement about how much to reveal.

> Holiday Care Service
> 2 Old Bank Chambers
> Station Road
> Horley
> Surrey RH6 9HW   (0293) 774535

The Malt House Trust

The Malt House Trust is a charity which offers short-stay accommodation (two or three weeks) for people in a crisis, for whatever reason. They welcome people with AIDS, although they have no facilities for people who need medical care. They also welcome people who have been on a rehabilitation programme, those who have been bereaved and those who care for others. The Trust can take ten people at a time, so there is privacy for those who want it. Accommodation is in a 'cosy, relaxed and homely environment' in a family house in a secluded part of a country town; the location is good as a base for walking and for a general rest. If you need a break as a carer the Trust may be the appropriate solution. Informal counselling is also available from members of the community who have skills in spiritual healing, counselling and social work. They have experience of both AIDS and bereavement. A week's stay, including all meals, costs £120. In some cases this can be paid by the DSS; if not, the Trust will do its best to find an alternative source of money, if necessary. Details from:

> The Malt House Trust
> The Malt House
> Church Street
> Uckfield
> East Sussex TN22 1BS   (0825) 61221

Appendices

Booklist

Living with AIDS: A Guide to Survival by People with AIDS – Frontliners, 1987; £9.95, free to people with ARC or AIDS; all proceeds go to help Frontliners – address on page 60.

Living with AIDS and HIV – David Miller, Macmillan Education, 1987, £7.95

Walking the Tightrope – Living Positively with AIDS, ARC and HIV – Jacqueline Hockings; £8 inc p+p from Gale Centre, Freepost, Loughton, Essex IG10 IBR

The Essential AIDS Fact Book – Paul Douglas and Laura Pinsky, Pocket Books, New York, 1989; £3.95

ABC of AIDS – edited by Michael Adler, British Medical Journal, 1987; £9.95

The Science of AIDS – Anthology, W H Freeman, Utah USA; $10.95

The Search for the Virus – Steve Connor and Sharon Kingman, revised and updated 1989, Penguin; £4.50

Taking Liberties: AIDS and Cultural Politics – edited by Erica Carter and Simon Watney, Serpents Tail 1989; £8.95

Matters of Life and Death: Women Speak about AIDS – edited by Ines Rieder and Patricia Ruppelt, Virago, 1989; £6.50

Wills and Probate – Consumers' Association,★ revised and updated 1989; £7.95

Make Your Will (England & Wales) – (Action pack) Consumers' Association,★ 1990; £7.95

How to Sort Out Someone's Will (England & Wales) – (Action pack) Consumers' Association,★ 1990; £7.95

★ Consumers' Association publications are available from bookshops or from: Consumers' Association, Castlemead, Gascoyne Way, Hertford SG14 1LH (p+p free).

Safer sex

The HIV virus has been found in semen, in women's vaginal juices and in menstrual blood. You cannot be infected unless the virus gets into your bloodstream. So there is no risk if any of these just come into contact with healthy unbroken skin. The virus can get in through the lining of the vagina, rectum or urethra, or through a wound. The biggest risk by far is through unprotected sexual intercourse – anal or vaginal sex without a condom. Some people avoid this risk altogether by not having penetrative sex. Sharing sex toys, and anything which may mean that blood or semen or other body fluids are exchanged, are also high risk activities. There may be small risks involved with oral sex – see below. Apart from these, sex is safe.

Condoms

You can reduce the risks a great deal – but not totally – by using a condom. The virus cannot pass through an unbroken condom. However, condoms can break, leak and, much more common, slip off. Make sure you know how to use condoms properly. All British Standard (BS 3704) Kitemarked brands now have detailed instructions. You should:

- always choose a Kitemarked brand or one which has been certified under a reputable national standard that you know about
- open the packet carefully, so as not to tear the condom
- squeeze the condom tip so no air is trapped inside
- unroll the condom on to the erect penis
- withdraw the penis after ejaculation, holding the condom rim to the base of the penis.

Practise using one with your eyes closed. Other points to remember:

- check the expiry date
- never use a condom twice
- never use one with oil-based lubricants like Vaseline, butter, handcream, olive oil, baby oil and so on – these will weaken the condom – in 15 minutes they can lose up to 92 per cent of their strength. Don't use spit. Instead, use water-based preparations such as KY Jelly, Duragel and Orthoforms.

Tests in laboratories have shown that the spermicide nonoxynol-9 can kill the HIV virus. Condoms with a spermicidal lubricant containing this will give you an extra layer of protection. Experts think that, providing sufficient lubricant is used, the risk of tearing a condom is no greater in anal intercourse than it is in vaginal intercourse.

Oral sex

It is is impossible to give a conclusive answer about how safe this is. Many experts believe there is little risk. Studies carried out so far have not shown oral sex as being a risk in itself, although sample sizes in these studies are sometimes too small to reveal small risks. There is also no reason to think that the virus should be able to get into your bloodstream through a healthy mouth – and stomach acids would probably kill it anyway. However, there is a theoretical risk that the virus in semen or vaginal juices could get into the bloodstream if you have ulcers or bleeding gums. There may be an increased risk during a woman's period. Some people use a condom or a 'dental dam' (a small square of latex bought from dental suppliers) during oral sex.

Number of partners

The important thing to remember is that it's not the number of people you have sex with that matters, but what you do. Unsafe sex with just one person could infect you. Some people who have an exclusive relationship with one person feel that they can have unsafe sex without risk. You have to both be sure that neither of you are infected and that you are totally faithful to each other.

Safer drugs

The following has been taken from *More Facts about AIDS for Drug Users* with the kind permission of the Terrence Higgins Trust.

Safer drugs

People who watch the way they use drugs stay healthier for longer than people who don't. This applies particularly to people infected with HIV. If you are antibody positive and continue to expose your body to further infections by fixing, sharing works and using contaminated street gear, you increase your chance of developing AIDS. So look at the way you use and see if you need to make changes. You can do several things, depending on what you want to do and what support and help is available.

You can stop sharing

- Always try to get your own set of works.
- Find a helpful local pharmacist or your nearest syringe exchange.
- Some areas are opening needle and syringe exchange schemes where you can get new works free.
- Use a clean set of works every time you fix.
- Keep your works safe so they can't be borrowed without your knowledge.
- Use your own spoon etc. for cooking up.
- Use clean water to mix with your gear.
- Dispose of your used works safely or through your exchange.

You can, if you have to share, clean your works

- Clean used equipment *immediately* it is used.
- Separate the needle, barrel and plunger and clean them in hot tap water and household detergent (washing-up liquid).
- Remove all traces of blood.
- Rinse the works thoroughly with clean water.
- Do the same with any spoons etc.
- After you have used the works, clean them in exactly the same way before anyone else uses them. Then get a new set of works as soon as possible.

NB: This method may kill any HIV present in the works. It will also help to stop blood clotting inside so that it can be flushed out effectively. However, it is always safer never to share cleaned works, even with partners or close friends.

You can stop fixing

- You can find lots of alternative ways of taking any drug which don't involve fixing or skin-popping.
- You can smoke or snort heroin.
- You can snort speed.
- You can drop pills (all opiate drugs can be found in oral form).
- You can freebase or snort coke.
- You can go over to oral substitutes like methadone (if you want to get a reliable supply you should approach a treatment centre or a doctor: it will mean fewer hassles in the long run).

You can stop using

- Don't be afraid to ask for help on this one: you don't have to go it alone.
- Find a local drugs agency to give you advice on self-help methods of coming off or other available treatment options.
- If you're using barbs or tranquillisers on a regular basis don't cut yourself down suddenly: reduce your daily dose very gradually.
- Explore the many self-help support groups like Narcotics Anonymous.
- Think about what you want in the long term: coming off isn't that difficult, staying off can be.
- Think about whom you're spending your time with: if your friends are users they may have their own problems and won't be able to give you much support.
- Consider the possibility of a rehab programme: you may need a break from the scene to get your life together.

Local helplines

There are over 70 local AIDS helplines which can give you up-to-date and local information.

We list the main helplines below, giving their telephone numbers and times when they are open. We are grateful to the *National AIDS Manual* for allowing us to extract this information which is up-to-date for September 1989. Please note that local services are constantly changing. To find the latest information contact the helpline nearest to you, the National AIDS Helpline (page 56), the London Lesbian and Gay Switchboard (which has a national service 01-837 7324), the Terrence Higgins Trust (page 57) or The Scottish AIDS Monitor (page 58). It may also be worth asking the Social Services department of your local authority for information.

LONDON

Brent	London Borough of Brent	01-961 5755	*24 hour helpline*
Ealing	Hounslow and Ealing AIDS Response Service	01-571 9191	*Monday, Wednesday, 6pm–9pm*
East London	London East AIDS Network	01-884 3344	*ask for reference number N510*
Enfield	AIDSline (Enfield)	01-366 9187	*office hours*
Hackney	Action on AIDS Team	01-739 8484(x4659)	*office hours*
Hammersmith and Fulham	Borough Social Services Department	01-748 3020 (x5147 area care teams; x4174 housing aid service)	*office hours*
Haringey	Haringey AIDS/HIV Forum	01-975 9700	*office hours*
Kensington and Chelsea	Kensington and Chelsea Social Services	01-937 5464 x2406	*office hours*

ENGLAND

Avon
Bath | Aled Richards Trust | (0225) 444347 | *Thursday 2.30pm to 4.30pm; 7.30pm to 9.30pm*

Bristol | Aled Richards Trust | (0272) 273436 | *Monday to Friday 7pm to 9pm*

Bedfordshire
Luton | Luton AIDS Community Support Unit | (0582) 404405 | *Tuesday, Thursday, Friday 7pm to 10pm*

Berkshire
Reading | Reading AIDS Line | (0734) 503377 | *Monday, Thursday 8pm to 10pm*

Slough | AIDS Support Group | (0753) 693050 | *Monday, Wednesday, Friday 8pm to 10pm*

Cambridgeshire
Cambridge | Cambridge AIDS Helpline | (0223) 69765 | *Tuesday, Wednesday, 7.30pm to 10pm, Saturday noon to 2pm*

Peterborough | Peterborough AIDS Helpline | (0733) 62334/311555 | *Tuesday, Thursday 7.30 pm to 9.30pm*

Cheshire
Chester | Chester and District AIDS Relief | (0244) 390300 | *Monday, Friday 7.30pm to 10pm*

Crewe | CADAR Crewe AIDS Helpline | (0270) 628938 | *Wednesday 8pm to 10pm*
Warrington | Warrington AIDS Line | (0925) 417134 | *Wednesday 7pm to 9pm*

Derbyshire
Derby | Derby AIDS Line | (0332) 290766 | *Monday to Friday 7pm to 9pm*
Thursday 2pm to 4pm, 7pm to 9pm

Devon
Exeter | Exeter AIDSline | (0392) 411600 | *Monday, Wednesday, Friday 7pm to 10pm*

Plymouth	Plymouth AIDS Support Group	(0752) 663609	*office hours*
Torquay	Torbay AIDS Group	(0803) 299266	*Friday 7.30pm to 10pm*
Dorset			
Bournemouth	Dorset Community Support Group	(0202) 292717	*Monday to Friday 8pm to 10pm*
Durham			
Bishop Auckland	AIDS Advice Centre	(0388) 602996	*Monday, Thursday 6pm to 9pm*
Essex			
Harlow	Harlow and District AIDS Support Group	(0279) 39199	*Sunday 4pm to 6pm*
Southend-on-Sea	Southend AIDSLINE	(0702) 460380	*Monday to Friday 6pm to 10 pm*
Gloucestershire			
Cheltenham	Gloucestershire AIDSline	(0242) 224666	*Monday, Wednesday 7pm to 9pm*
Greater Manchester			
Manchester	Manchester AIDSline	(061) 228 1617	*Monday to Friday 7pm to 10pm*
Hampshire			
Portsmouth	Portsmouth AIDSLINE	(0705) 672666	*Thursday 7.30pm to 10pm*
Southampton	Solent AIDS Line	(0703) 637363	*Tuesday, Thursday, Friday 7.30pm to 10pm*
	AIDSline Southampton	(0703) 339467	*Friday 7.30pm to 10pm*
Hereford & Worcester			
Kidderminster	Kidderminster AIDS Counselling line	(0562) 66766	*Monday to Friday 9am to 12.30pm, 2pm to 4pm*

Hertfordshire

Hemel Hempstead	The Crescent – HIV/AIDS Information and Counselling Centre	(0442) 42042	*Monday 7pm to 9.30pm*
St Albans	The Crescent – HIV/AIDS Information and Counselling Centre	(0727) 44230	*Monday 7pm to 9.30pm*
		(0727) 42532	*Monday to Thurdays 10am to 4pm*
Stevenage	North Herts AIDS Helpline	(0438) 740270	*Tuesday, Thursday 7.30pm to 10pm*

Humberside

Beverley	AIDSACTION North Humberside	(0482) 870451	*Monday, Thursday, Saturday 10am to 2pm; Tuesday, Thursday 7pm to 9pm; Wednesday, Sunday 7pm to 10pm; Friday 9pm to 1 am*
Bridlington	AIDSACTION North Humberside	(0262) 400440	*Monday, Thursday, Saturday 10am to 2pm; Tuesday, Thursday 7pm to 9pm; Wednesday, Sunday 7pm to 10pm; Friday 9pm to 1am*
Grimsby	Grimsby AIDSline	(0472) 240840	*Monday, Thursday 7.30pm to 9.30pm*
Hull	AIDSACTION North Humberside	(0482) 27060	*Monday, Thursday, Saturday 10am to 2pm; Tuesday, Thursday 7pm to 9pm; Wednesday, Sunday 7pm to 10pm; Friday 9pm to 1 am*

Kent

Dartford	AIDS Support Cooperative	(0322) 92610	*Monday to Friday 8.45 am to 5pm*

Folkestone	Folkestone AIDS Helpline	(0303) 41444	*Monday, Friday, Saturday, Sunday 7pm to 10pm*
Margate	East Kent AIDS Helpline	(0843) 298610	*Monday to Friday 7pm to 10pm*
Medway	AIDS Support Cooperative	(0634) 830000 x3532	*Monday to Friday 8.45am to 5pm*

Lancashire

| Burnley | Burnley AIDS Helpline | (0282) 831101 | *Friday 7.30pm to 9.30pm* |
| Lancaster | North Lancs and South Cumbria AIDS line | (0524) 841011 | *Monday 7pm to 10pm* |

Leicestershire

| Leicester | Leicester Lesbian and Gayline | (0533) 550667 | *Monday to Friday 7.30pm to 10.30pm* |
| | Leicestershire AIDS Support Services | (0533) 549922 (x6429) | *Monday to Friday 9am to 5pm* |

Lincolnshire

Boston	Boston AIDS Helpline	(0205) 354462	*Monday, Tuesday 9.15 am to 10.15am; Thursday 11.15pm to 1.15 am*
Grantham	Grantham AIDS Helpline	(0476) 60192	*Monday, Friday 9am to 10am; Wednesday 1.30pm to 3pm*
Lincoln	Lincoln AIDS Helpline	(0522) 545371	*Monday, Wednesday 5pm to 7pm*

Merseyside

| Liverpool | Merseyside AIDS Support Group | (051) 709 9000 | *Monday, Wednesday, Friday 7pm to 10pm* |

Norfolk

| Norwich | Norwich AIDS Helpline | (0603) 615816 | *Thursday 8pm to 10pm* |
| Waveney | Waveney and Great Yarmouth AIDS Helpline | (0502) 501509 | *Friday 6pm to 8pm* |

Northamptonshire			
Northampton	AIDS Counselling and Education Service	(0604) 28999	*Monday to Friday 9am to 7pm*
North Yorkshire			
Harrogate	AIDS Concern North Yorkshire	(0423) 505222	*Monday, Thursday 7pm to 9pm*
Nottinghamshire			
Mansfield	Mansfield AIDS Helpline	(0623) 642814	*Monday 7pm to 9pm*
Nottingham	Nottingham AIDS Information Project	(0602) 585526	*Monday, Thursday 7pm to 10pm*
Oxfordshire			
Oxford	OXAIDS	(0865) 728817	*Sunday, Monday, Wednesday, Friday 6pm to 8pm*
Shropshire			
Shrewsbury	Shrewsbury AIDS Helpline	(0743) 232748	*Monday, Wednesday, Thursday 2pm to 5pm*
South Yorkshire			
Sheffield	Sheffield AIDSline	(0800) 844334	*Monday to Friday 7pm to 10pm*
Staffordshire			
Stafford	Mid-Staffordshire AIDSline	(0785) 57731	*Monday to Friday 9am to 5pm*
Suffolk			
Bury St Edmunds	Bury St Edmunds AIDSline	(0284) 702544 (x2185) (0284) 89372	*office hours* *24 hours*
Ipswich	Ipswich AIDSline	(0473) 232007	*Tuesday, Friday, 7.30pm to 10pm*
Lowestoft	Waveney and Great Yarmouth AIDS Helpline	(0493) 501509	*Friday, 6pm to 8pm*

Surrey
Guildford | SEAL (Surrey & East Hants AIDS Helpline) | (0483) 300150 | *Tuesday, Wednesday, Friday 8pm to 10pm*

Sussex
Brighton | Sussex AIDS Centre & Helpline | (0273) 571660 | *Monday to Friday, 8pm to 10pm*

Hastings | Hastings and Rother AIDS Support Society | (0424) 429901 | *Monday to Friday 2.30pm to 4.30pm*

Eastbourne | Eastbourne AIDS Helpline | (0323) 20322 | *Monday to Friday 10am to 1pm*

| | (042) 693 3008 | *Bleep service 24 hours*

Tyne & Wear
Newcastle upon Tyne | Community Support Centre | (091) 273 0197 | *office hours*

| Body Positive North East | (091) 232 2855 | *Monday to Friday 10am to 5pm*

Sunderland | District Health Authority AIDSline | (091) 522 6045 | *office hours*

Warwickshire
Rugby | Rugby AIDS Helpline | (0788) 540160 | *office hours*

West Midlands
Walsall | Walsall AIDSline | (0922) 644853 | *Monday to Friday 10am to 4pm*

West Midlands | AIDS Line West Midlands | (021) 622 1511 | *Monday to Friday 7.30pm to 10pm*

Wiltshire
Salisbury | Salisbury AIDS Helpline | (0722) 411064 | *Wednesday 7pm to 9pm; Thursday 6pm to 8pm*

West Yorkshire
Bradford | Pennine AIDS Link | (0274) 732939 | *Monday to Thursday 7.30pm to 9.30pm*

Huddersfield | Kirklees Helpline | (0484) 434825 | *Monday to Sunday 7pm to 11pm*

| Leeds | Leeds AIDS Advice | (0532) 444209 | *Monday to Friday 7pm to 9pm* |

SCOTLAND

Aberdeen	Grampian AIDS Line	(0224) 574000	*answerphone directory*
Edinburgh	Scottish AIDS Monitor	(0345) 090966	*Monday to Friday 7.30pm to 10pm*
Glasgow	Scottish AIDS Monitor	(0345) 090966	*Monday to Friday 7.30pm to 10pm*

WALES

Dyfed

| Haverfordwest | Dyfed AIDS Helpline | (0437) 762009 | *Monday, Friday 8pm to 10pm* |

Gwent

| Newport | Gwent AIDS Advice Line | (0633) 422532 | *Monday to Friday 9am to 5pm, Tuesdays until 8pm* |
| | Gwent AIDS Helpline | (0633) 841901 | *Monday to Friday, 8.30am to 4pm* |

Gwynedd

| Llandudno | AIDS Care North Wales | (0492) 860569 | *Thursday 7pm to 10pm* |

Powys

| Brecon | Powys AIDS Line Services (PALS) | (0597) 4200 | *Wednesday, Saturday, 8pm to 11pm* |
| | Welsh speaking | (0597) 2800 | *Wednesday, Saturday, 8pm to 11pm* |

South Glamorgan

| Cardiff | Cardiff AIDS Helpline | (0222) 223443 | *Monday to Friday 7pm to 10pm* |

West Glamorgan
Swansea | Swansea AIDS Helpline | (0792) 456303 | *Thursday 3pm to 8pm*

NORTHERN IRELAND

Belfast | AIDS Helpline | (0232) 326117 | *Monday, Wednesday, Friday 7.30pm to 10pm; Saturday 2pm to 5pm*

CHANNEL ISLANDS

Jersey | Jersey AIDS Relief Group | (0534) 58886 | *Daily 6pm to 10pm*

Feedback

Information in this book was correct at the time of going to press in the autumn of 1989.

Please tell us if you know of any other sources of help, information or services that have been set up since then. Your experiences about how easy or difficult it has been to get any help you have needed would also be most welcome, as are your opinions of any of the organisations you have approached.

We would also be grateful for your views – good or bad – about this book, and for any ideas about how any similar book could be improved or developed in the future.

Research Institute for Consumer Affairs
2 Marylebone Road
London NW1 4DX

Index

ABC of Aids   289
ACAS (Advisory, Conciliation and
    Arbitration Service)   101
acceptance   210
Access to Medical Reports Act   97
*Access to the Underground: a Guide for
    Elderly and Disabled People*   138
accommodation, finding   121
accommodation, temporary   124
Accommodation Team, Lothian
    Regional Council   130
ACET (AIDS, Care, Education and
    Training)   65; grants 176, 264
Acquired Immunodeficiency Syndrome
    see AIDS
ACT-UP (Aids Coalition to Unleash
    Power)   78
acupuncture   199
acute infection   15
acyclovir   191
adaptations   135
Additional Tax Allowance   161
ADFAM National   242
Advisory Legal Bureau on AIDS *see*
    ALBA
Advisory, Conciliation and Arbitration
    Service *see* ACAS
AIDS   195
AIDS (Acquired Immunodeficiency
    Syndrome)   12

AIDS AHEAD   177
AIDS and Housing Project   126
AIDS Care Education and Training *see*
    ACET
AIDS Coalition to Unleash Power *see*
    ACT-UP
AIDS dementia *see* dementia
Aids Education and Research Trust *see*
    AVERT
AIDS Helpline (Northern Ireland)   58
AIDS Information   194
AIDS Mastery   199
AIDS Newsletter   195
AIDS Treatment News   195
AIDS-related-complex *see* ARC
AIDS—the Facts for Working Girls   107
*AIDS/HIV Experimental Treatment
    Directory*   195
*AIDS: Some Questions and Answers.
    Facts for Teachers, Lecturers and
    Youth Workers*   222
Air Transport Users' Committee   141
AL-721   192, 193, 199
ALBA (Advisory Legal Bureau on
    AIDS)   107
Albany Trust Counselling   205
Aled Richards Trust   61; grants 177
Alexander Technique   273
All Wales Drugline   240
alpha-interferon   191, 192

ambulance services   140
American Foundation for AIDS
    Research   195
amphotericin   187, 189
ampligen   192
Ananda Network   265
Angel Project (Inner City Action on
    Drugs)   130
anti-depressants   275
anti-HIV treatment   192
antibody positive   15
appearance, worries about   41
ARC (AIDS-related-complex)   16
Association of British Insurers   96
Association of Continence
    Advisors   117
Association of Crossroads Care
    Attendant Schemes   283
ATN Publications   196
Attendance Allowance   155
autogenic training   199
AVERT (Aids Education and Research
    Trust)   222
AZT *see* zidovudine

Bactrim   186
BACUP   73
Badger's Parting Gifts   218
Bailey Brothers & Swinfen Ltd   194
bathing attendants   50

bed and breakfast accommodation   124
bedsores *see* pressure sores
benefits, booklets   172
benefits, factsheet   174
benefits, guides   172
bereavement   255
birth   214
Black HIV and AIDS Network   59
Blackliners   59
Blind Persons Income Tax
    Allowance   155
Bloomsbury Community Care
    Team   62
board and lodging allowances   167
Body Positive   59; grants   178, 278
Body Positive Centre   66
BP News   59
breastfeeding   214
British Association for Counselling   86
British Association of
    Psychotherapists   88
British Dental Association   35
British Humanist Association   252
British Library   200
British Medical Association   97
British Medical Journal   195
British Psychological Society   89
British Rail and Disabled Travellers   142
British Red Cross Society   75
Brook Advisory Centres   90
Buddhist Hospice Trust   265
buddy schemes   68
budgeting loan   171
Bureau of Hygiene and Tropical
    Diseases   194, 195
burial   252

campylobacter enteritis   188
Cancer Link   74
cancer organisations   73
Cancer Relief (Macmillan Fund)   52
CARA (Care and Resources for People
    Affected by AIDS/HIV)   264
Care and Resources for People Affected
    by AIDS/HIV *see* CARA

care at home   283
care attendant schemes   283
care away from home   285
*Care in the Air—Advice for Handicapped
    Travellers*   141
Carematch   286
Carer's Premium   157, 165, 167
Carers' National Association   279
carers, caring for   267
caring, general   19
Caring and Sharing Together in
    Lothian and Edinburgh *see*
    CASTLE
Caring Together   279
CASTLE (Caring and Sharing
    Together in Lothian and
    Edinburgh)   278
Catholic AIDS Link   266
Cave House   128
CD4   192, 193
Centers for Disease Control   15
Central Office of the Industrial
    Tribunals   100
Central Services Agency List   49
cerebral toxoplasmosis   189
Charities Digest   176
CHART (Customers helping AIDS
    relief trust)   178
Chelsea Pastoral Foundation   88
chemotherapy   191
Child Benefit   161
Child Poverty Action Group   174
children   213
*Children at School and Problems Related to
    AIDS*   222
Children Bill   219
children, caring for   215
Christian Action on AIDS   264
Citizens Advice Bureau   48, 80
City Roads (Crisis Intervention)   236
Civil Legal Aid   103
Clinic 8, AIDS Counselling Unit   85
clinical psychology   89
clinical trials   196
CMV (cytomegalovirus)   188, 189

Co-trimoxazole   186
*Code of Professional Conduct for the
    Nurse*   52
Cold Weather Payment   171
community care aides   54
Community Care Grant   171
Community Charge, rebates   164
community drug teams   232
Community Health Council   48, 80
community psychiatric nurses   51
Community Support Centre,
    Newcastle   65
Compassionate Friends   261
complaining   79
complementary medicine   199
Complementary Medicine Index   200
compulsory care   219
concessionary fare scheme   154
condoms   291
confidentiality   144
confidentiality, medical   52
constructive dismissal   101
Consumers' Association   105
continence adviser   117
corticosteroids   187
cosmetic camouflage   75, 190
Council for Voluntary Service   48, 74
council housing   125
Council of Social Service   74
counselling   83
*Counselling and Psychotherapy Resources
    Directory*   86
Court of Protection   95
cremation   252
Criminal Injuries Compensation
    Board   163
crisis loan   168, 172
Crossroads *see* Association of
    Crossroads Care Attendant
    Schemes
Crossroads Scotland   284
CRUSAID   178
CRUSE   261
cryptococcal meningitis   189
cryptosporidiosis   188

Current AIDS Literature   194
Current Science Ltd   195
cytomegalovirus (CMV)   188, 189

David Manley Fund   178
David Miller   23
day centres   66
day hospitals   285
DDU *see* drug dependency units
death, facing   46
death certificate   247
death, what to do when someone
    dies   247
dementia   41, 190
dental treatment, free   160
dentists   35
Department of Education and
    Science   217, 222
Department of Employment   99
Department of Social Security   143
Department of Social Security,
    freephone enquiry service   143
Department of the Environment   136
Department of Transport   137
depression   41
Depressives Associated   276
dextran sulphate   192
diagnosis, after   29
Dial-a-Ride   138
diarrhoea   188
dideoxycytidine   192
dideoxyinosine   192
*Directory of Airline Facilities for Disabled
    People*   141
*Directory of Counselling Services in
    Scotland*   87
Directory of Grant-Making Trusts   176
*Directory of Grant-Making Trusts and
    Organisations in Scotland*   176
Disability Alliance ERA   174
Disability Premium   166
Disability Rights Handbook   174
Disabled Living Foundation   117
Disabled Person's Railcard   141, 154
Disablement Income Group   144

dismissal   99
district committees   49
district nurses   50
domiciliary care aides   54
donor insemination   14
Door to Door   137
drop in centres   67
drug:
    advice agencies   230
    dependency units   231
    laws   243
    substitutes   236
    users   225
drugs, self help and community
    groups   239
dry skin   191
DSS Leaflet Unit   173
duty of care   53

early intervention   193
egg yolk therapy *see* AL-721
Emergency Housing Office   123
employment   98
Enduring Power of Attorney   94
enema   118
escorts:
    British Red Cross   75
    WRVS   76
ethics committee   196
eviction   133
exercise   274

FACTS (Foundation for AIDS
    Counselling Treatment and
    Support)   194
Families Anonymous   242
families, caring for   203
Family Credit   169
Family Fund   162
Family Practitioners Committee   49,
    81
Family Support Network   277
family therapy   90
Fansidar   187
fares, concessionary   154

Fellowship of Depressives
    Anonymous   276
FLAGS (Family Life AIDS
    Groups)   128
fluconazole   187, 189
flucytosine   189
Foscarnet   189
Foundation for AIDS Counselling
    Treatment and Support *see* FACTS
Freefone Drug Problems   240
Friends support group   278
Frontiers   60
Frontliners   60; grants 179
funeral:
    ceremonies   251
    directors   250
    expenses   158
    payment   170
funerals   250

ganciclovir   189
Gay Bereavement Project   105, 262
Gay Legal Advice *see* GLAD
General Dental Council   81
General Medical Council   79
general practitioner *see* GP
General Synod of the Church of
    England   265
giardiasis   188
GLAD (Gay Legal Advice)   107
GP (general practitioner)   48; and
    drugs 231
GPs, changing   50
Green Form Scheme   103
grieving   256
guardianship   220
*Guide to Grants for Individuals in
    Need*   176
Guild of Social Welfare   74

haemophilia   245
haemophilia centres   246
Haemophilia Society   245
haemophilia, single and weekly
    payments   162

Hammersmith and Fulham Shared Housing   127
HART (Holistic AIDS Research Trust)   201
health district   49
Health Education Unit   238
Health Literature Line   56
Health Service Commissioner (Ombudsman)   80
health visitors   50
Healthline   276
help, domestic, WRVS   76
Help the Hospices   71
helper cells   69
herpes   191
herpes simplex   191
herpes zoster   191
HIV (Human Immunodeficiency Virus)   12
HIV clinics   31
HIV, You and the Law   107
HIV-positive   15
Holiday Care Service   286
holidays   286
Holistic AIDS Research Trust *see* HART
Holistic Health Group   61
home care aides   54
home care teams   62
home helps   54
home nursing, British Red Cross   75, 109
Home Support Team, St Mary's Hospital   62
home support teams *see* home care teams
Homeless Persons' Unit   123
homelessness   122
homeopathy   199
Hospice Information Service   71
hospices   69
hospital, allowances   168
hostels   125
housing   121
Housing Act, 1985   122, 131

housing adaptations   55, 135
Housing Advice Centre   126
Housing Advice Switchboard   129
Housing Aid Centres   130
Housing and HIV Infection   123, 124
housing associations   125
Housing Benefit   166
Housing Booklet No 14: A Guide to Home Improvement Grants   136
Housing Corporation   125
housing law   131
How to Sort Out Someone's Will   105, 290
Humanist Funeral Ceremonies   252
human immunodeficiency virus *see* HIV
hygiene, domestic   211
hygiene, nursing   119

IATA   141
Immunity   107
Implications of AIDS for Children in Care   223
improvement grants   136
INCAD (Incapacitated Passengers Handling Advice)   140
Incapacitated Passengers Air Travel Guide   141
Incapacitated Passengers Handling Advice *see* INCAD
Incapacity Pension   153
Income Support   165
incontinence   117
Independent Living Fund   156
Industrial Injuries Disablement Benefit   163
industrial tribunals   99, 100
infection:
  children   214
  risks of   12, 211, 214
  stages of   15
Inheritance Act   105
Inner City Action on Drugs *see* Angel Project
Institute for Complementary Medicine   200

Institute for the Study of Drug Dependence *see* ISDD
Institute of Family Therapy   90
Insurance Ombudsman Bureau   98
Interfaith Group   263
intermediate grant *see* improvement grant
Invalid Care Allowance   157
Invalidity Benefit   150
ISDD (Institute for the Study of Drug Dependence)   240

Jewish AIDS Trust   266
Jewish Lesbian and Gay Helpline   266
Joseph Rowntree Memorial Trust   162

Kaposi's sarcoma   11, 43, 187, 190
Keeping Fit While Caring   274
Ketoconazole   187
Kings Fund Informal Caring Programme   280
Kobler Centre   60, 66
KS *see* Kaposi's sarcoma
Kubler-Ross, Elisabeth   256

LAGER (Lesbian and Gay Employment Rights)   103
Lancet, The   195
Landmark   66
Lantern Trust   279
laundry services   55
law centres   107
LEAN (London East AIDS Network)   179
Legal Advice and Assistance Scheme *see* Green Form Scheme
Legal Aid   103
legal matters   93
Leicestershire AIDS Support Services   378
Lesbian and Gay Christian Movement   265
Lesbian and Gay Employment Rights *see* LAGER
Let's Face It   43

libraries 48
life insurance 95
Lifeskills 274
Lions Club International Secretariat 77
live-in help 284
live-in help, National Insurance 285
living with AIDS 21
Living with AIDS and HIV 23, 289
Living with AIDS: A Guide to Survival by People with AIDS 60, 289
local AIDS helplines 295
Local Authority Association's Working Group on AIDS 123
local health council 49
London Dial-a-Ride Users' Association 139
London East AIDS Network *see* LEAN
London Housing Aid Centre *see* SHAC
London Lesbian and Gay Centre 60, 85
London Lesbian and Gay Switchboard 107, 209, 295
London Lighthouse 71
  day centre 67
  home support service 63
London Regional Transport 138
London Taxicard scheme 139, 154
Lothian Regional Council's Supported Accommodation Team AIDS 130
Lovers' Support Group 278
low income 164

MacFarlane Trust 162, 179
Macmillan Fund 52; grants 180
Macmillan nurses 50
MAI *see* tuberculosis
Mainliners grants 180, 239
Make Your Will 105, 290
Malcolm Sargent Cancer Fund 180
Malt House Trust 287
Manchester Interfaith Group 264
Marie Curie Cancer Care 52; grants 181, 284, 286
massage 199, 273
Maternity Allowance 160

Maternity Payment 161, 171
Matters of Life and Death: Women Speak about AIDS 290
Meals on Wheels 55
Medical Directory 49
Medical Information Service, British Library 200
medical loan service, British Red Cross 75
member of parliament 81
meningitis 189
Mental Welfare Commission for Scotland 94
methadone 236
Metropolitan Community Church 266
Middlesex Hospital 62
Mildmay Mission Hospital 72
MIND (National Association for Mental Health) 275
Minnesota Method 233
Mobility Allowance 153
molluscum contagiosum 191
Monument Trust 181
mortgages 96
mortgages, difficulty paying 134
mouth ulcers 188

Narcotics Anonymous 233, 240
National Advisory Unit 139
National AIDS Helpline 56
National AIDS Manual 28, 49, 56, 201
National AIDS Trust 78
National Association for Mental Health *see* MIND
National Association of Funeral Directors 249, 250
National Association of Round Tables 76
National Association of Young People's Counselling and Advisory Services *see* NAYPCAS
National Childbirth Trust 222
National Childminding Association 223

National Council for Voluntary Organisations *see* NCVO
National Federation of Housing Associations 126
National Foster Care Association 223
National Health Service 48, 79
National Secular Society 252
National Tranquilliser Advice Centre *see* TRANX
National Welfare Benefits Handbook 174
NAYPCAS (National Association of Young People's Counselling and Advisory Services) 91, 241
NCVO (National Council for Voluntary Organisations) 74
needle and syringe exchanges 238
Network of Voluntary Organisations in AIDS/HIV *see* NOVOAH
New Scientist 195
Newcastle community support team 64
NHS charges, free 169
Nightlights 63
nightshelters 124
Northern Ireland Association for Counselling 87
Northern Ireland Regional Drug Unit 240
Notes on Incontinence 117
NOVOAH (Network of Voluntary Organisations in AIDS/HIV) 78
nurseries 217
nursing aids 51
nursing auxiliaries 50
nursing homes, allowances 168
nystatin 187

obsessional thoughts 45
Occupational Sick Pay 149
occupational therapists (OTs) 51, 54
oesophageal candida 188
Ombudsman, health *see* Health Service Commissioner
Ombudsman, Insurance 98
Ombudsman, Parliamentary 81

On Death and Dying 256
Oncology Information Service 194
One Parent Benefit 161
opportunistic infections 16
OPUS (Organisation for Parents Under
    Stress) 243
oral candida (thrush) 187
oral sex 291
Orange Badge Parking Scheme 154
Organisation for Parents Under Stress
    see OPUS
OTs *see* occupational therapists
OXAIDS 65; grants 181

PACE (Project for Advice, Counselling
    and Education) 85
Parentline-OPUS 91
Parents' Enquiry 210
partners, caring for 203
Patients' Association 81
PCP (pneumocystis carinii
    pneumonia) 186
Pentamidine 187
persistent generalised lymphadenopathy
    see PGL
PGL (persistent generalised
    lymphadenopathy) 16
Phoenix House 235
phosphonoformate 189
Physical Fitness 274
physiotherapists 51
Piccadilly Advice Centre 129
Pink Form Scheme *see* Green Form
    Scheme
placebo 196, 200
playgroups 217
pneumocystis carinii pneumonia *see*
    PCP
poll tax *see* Community Charge
Positive Help 64
Positive Partners 61
Positive Women in Scotland 222
Positively Close 61
Positively Women, childrens'
    fund 181, 221, 239
post-mortem 248

Power of Attorney 93
pregnancy 213
prejudice 209
prescriptions, free 155, 160
pressure sores 115, 191
Project for Advice, Counselling and
    Education *see* PACE
Psychology Department, St Mary's
    Hospital 86
psychotherapy 88
Pyrimethamine 189

RADAR (Royal Association for
    Disability and Rehabilitation) 142
radiotherapy 190
Rationalist Press Association 252
Reaching Out 265
redundancy 102
Register of Chartered Psychologists 89
registering a death 248
rehabilitation centres 232
Relate (National Marriage
    Guidance) 90
relaxation 199, 274
Relaxation for Living 274
RELEASE 241
religious groups 263
religious support 263
Rent Act 131
repatriation 249
Research Council for Complementary
    Medicine 200
resettlement units 124
residential care homes, allowances 168
residential homes 168
respite care 282
retrovir *see* zidovudine
*Rights Guide to Non-Means Tested
    Benefits* 174
Road Tax 154
ROMA 235
Rotary Clubs (Rotary International in
    Great Britain and Northern
    Ireland) 76
Round Tables *see* National Association
    of Round Tables

Royal Association for Disability and
    Rehabilitation *see* RADAR
Ruchill Hospital 64
rural community council 74

safer drug use 292
safer sex 290
salmonellosis 188
Salvation Army 182
SAM (Scottish AIDS Monitor) 58,
    grants 182
Samaritans 243, 276
schools 217
Science of AIDS 289
Scientific American 195
SCODA (Standing Conference on
    Drug Abuse) 241
Scottish AIDS Monitor *see* SAM
Scottish Association for
    Counselling 87
Scottish Drugs Forum 240, 241
Scottish Education Department 217
Scottish Homes 125
Scottish Marriage Guidance
    Council 90
Search for the Virus 289
seborrhoeic dermatitis 191
self-help groups 59
Septrin 186
seroconversion 15
seropositive 15
Severe Disability Premium 157
Severe Disablement Allowance 151
sex and drugs 229
sex and transmission of HIV 12, 290
sex, problems with 205, 229
Sexual and Personal Relationships of
    People with a Disability *see* SPOD
sexually transmitted disease clinics *see*
    STD clinics
SHAC (London Housing Aid
    Centre) 129
Shelter (National Campaign for the
    Homeless) 130
shingles 191
Sickness Benefit 149

sitting services 283
skin rashes see symptoms, skin
sleeping 273
Social Care Resource Centre 126, 265
Social Fund 170
Social Security see Department of Social
    Security
Social Security benefit leaflets 172
social workers 53
Society of Teachers of the Alexander
    Technique 273
South Place Ethical Society 252
South West Thames Regional Drug
    Dependence and Research
    Unit 241
spastic paraparaesis 190
Special Needs Housing Advisory
    Service 126
spectacles, vouchers for 165, 169
SPOD (Sexual and Personal
    Relationships of People with a
    Disability) 206
St John Ambulance 139
St John's Housing Association 127
St Mary's Hospital AIDS
    counselling 86
St Mungo Community Trust 128
St Mungo FLAGS (Family Life AIDS
    Groups) 128
Standard Grant 136
Standing Conference on Drug Abuse
    see SCODA
Statutory Instrument No 1450 193
Statutory Maternity Pay 160
Statutory Sick Pay 148
STD clinics 31
stigma 45
street agencies 230
stress 41, 199, 271
Strutton Housing Association 127
sulphadiazine 189
support groups, THT 57;
    Body Positive 60
suppositories 118
Sussex AIDS Centre and Helpline 63,
    67

Sussex AIDS Centre and Helpline day
    centre 67
Sussex AIDS Centre and Helpline home
    care support team 63
symptoms:
    constitutional 186
    gastrointestinal 187
    general 16, 185
    in children 215
    neurological 190
    respiratory 186
    skin 190

T-Helper cells 12
TACADE (Teachers Advisory Council
    on Alcohol and Drug
    Education) 242
Taking a Break 280, 285
Taking Liberties: AIDS and Cultural
    Politics 290
taking time off 280
taxis 139
Teachers Advisory Council on
    Alcohol and Drug Education
    see TACADE
Telling your Parents 210
temporary accommodation 124
tenancy 131
tenancy, harassment 133
tenancy, inheriting 134
Terrence Higgins Trust (THT) 57;
    grants 182
test for HIV 16, 203; children 214
The Essential AIDS Fact Book 289
The Implications of AIDS for Children in
    Care 223
The Medicines Order 1971 193
therapeutic communities 232
Threshold Housing Advice
    Centre 130
thrush see oral candida
THT see Terrence Higgins Trust
tinea 191
toilets, special 142
toxoplasma gondii 189
tranquillisers 275

Trans Pennine Housing Consortium
    (TPHC) 129
transmission:
    birth 14
    blood 13
    caring and nursing 14
    donor insemination 14
    kissing 14
    sharing a household 14
transport:
    air 140
    ambulance, British Red Cross 75,
        139
    bus 137
    local 137
    social services 140
    taxi 139
    train 141
    underground 137
    volunteers 139
TRANX (National Tranquilliser
    Advice Centre) 275
Travel-Care 140
trials see clinical trials
Trimethoprim 187
Tripscope 142
tuberculosis 187
Turning Point 235, 242

ulcerative gingivitis 188
unemployed 147
Unemployment Benefit 147
unfair dismissal 99
United Kingdom Central Council for
    Nursing, Midwifery and Health
    Visiting 53
vaccinations 204, 216
Vehicle Excise Duty (Road Tax) 154
vesting property 95
voluntary care 220
Voluntary Council for Handicapped
    Children 223
voluntary organisations, general 74

Waverley Care Trust 73
weight loss 188

welfare benefit leaflets   172
welfare benefit review   172
welfare benefits   143
welfare benefits index   145
welfare benefits, collecting   175
Westminster Hospital   63
Westminster Pastoral Foundation   88
Westminster Social Services Home Care
    Team   63
What is homosexuality?   210

What to Do When Someone Dies   254
When Uncle Bob Died   218
Which benefit?   173
Who Minds about AIDS?   223
Widow's Additional Pension   159
Widow's Benefits   158
Widow's Bereavement Allowance   158
Widow's Payment   158
Widow's Pension   159
Widowed Mother's Allowance   159

Wills   104
Wills and Probate   105, 290
Women's Royal Voluntary Service *see*
    WRVS
wrongful dismissal   102
WRVS   76

Your Rights at Work   107

zidovudine   189, 190, 191, 192, 193, 215